Blooming in December: Psychodynamic Psychotherapy with Older Adults

This book covers the essentials of psychotherapeutic work with older adults, discussing how contemporary psychodynamic thought can be applied clinically to engage the older patient in psychotherapeutic work of depth and meaning, work that not only relieves suffering but also promotes growth.

It describes the way the difficulties accompanying older age can affect psychological functioning and it examines the unique psychotherapeutic needs of this age group. Using clinical vignettes for illustrative purposes, it explores the psychotherapeutic challenges, tasks, techniques, and accomplishments involved in the treatment of older adults. Topics discussed include the reemergence of earlier developmental challenges; the concurrent treatment of late life and revived early trauma; transference and countertransference; the functions of developing an enriched life narrative in restoring the self; existential issues; and mourning. Throughout, the focus is on what psychotherapy can do to help.

The demand for mental health services for older adults is growing alongside increasing life spans, but the psychodynamic literature has neglected this population. *Blooming in December: Psychodynamic Psychotherapy with Older Adults* fills this gap, offering a clear guide to effective work with older adults for all psychotherapists and psychoanalysts.

Amy Schaffer, PhD, is a faculty member and supervisor at the Institute for Contemporary Psychotherapy and the Psychoanalytic Psychotherapy Study Center. A psychologist/psychoanalyst in private practice, she also has a background in psychological research and psychodrama in mental health settings. She has worked with older adults in her practice for 40 years.

Psychoanalysis in a New Key Book Series
Series Editor: Donnel Stern

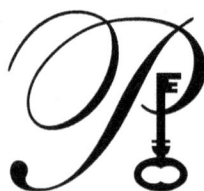

When music is played in a new key, the melody does not change, but the notes that make up the composition do: change in the context of continuity, continuity that perseveres through change. Psychoanalysis in a New Key publishes books that share the aims psychoanalysts have always had, but that approach them differently. The books in the series are not expected to advance any particular theoretical agenda, although to this date most have been written by analysts from the Interpersonal and Relational orientations.

The most important contribution of a psychoanalytic book is the communication of something that nudges the reader's grasp of clinical theory and practice in an unexpected direction. Psychoanalysis in a New Key creates a deliberate focus on innovative and unsettling clinical thinking. Because that kind of thinking is encouraged by exploration of the sometimes surprising contributions to psychoanalysis of ideas and findings from other fields, Psychoanalysis in a New Key particularly encourages interdisciplinary studies. Books in the series have married psychoanalysis with dissociation, trauma theory, sociology, and criminology. The series is open to the consideration of studies examining the relationship between psychoanalysis and any other field – for instance, biology, literary and art criticism, philosophy, systems theory, anthropology, and political theory.

But innovation also takes place within the boundaries of psychoanalysis, and Psychoanalysis in a New Key therefore also presents work that reformulates thought and practice without leaving the precincts of the field. Books in the series focus, for example, on the significance of personal values in psychoanalytic practice, on the complex interrelationship between the analyst's clinical work and personal life, on the consequences for the clinical situation when patient and analyst are from different cultures, and on the need for psychoanalysts to accept the degree to which they knowingly satisfy their own wishes during treatment hours, often to the patient's detriment.

A full list of all titles in this series is available at: www.routledge.com/series/LEAPNKBS

"This wise, readable book finally rectifies the psychoanalytic community's shameful inattention to – and devaluation of – psychotherapy with aging patients. As we boomers confront a life phase for which neither the dominant culture nor our countercultural ideologies prepared us, we look to psychotherapists for help (after all, one of our generation's achievements was to destigmatize therapy). But before Schaffer's contribution, otherwise well-trained psychoanalytic clinicians were ill-equipped to help us face the challenges, losses, and insults of getting old – not to mention its gratifications and rewards. All therapists should read this scholarly, insightful, clinically invaluable work."

– **Nancy McWilliams, PhD, ABPP**, Rutgers University Graduate School of Applied & Professional Psychology

"Amy Schaffer's new book is a distinctive contribution to a frequently overlooked area – working psychoanalytically with the older adult. Schaffer convincingly challenges the agism inherent in the assumption that older patients are unable to engage in deep psychoanalytic work. She points to the limitations inherent in aging – choices have been made and cannot be un-made – yet reminds us of how much can nevertheless be done. Addressing a range of issues relevant to clinical work in general and aging in particular, Schaffer's book is rich with clinical experience and wisdom. A must-read for all of us."

– **Joyce Slochower, PhD,** NYU Postdoctoral Program

"This seminal book is a welcome arrival that counters the psychoanalytic bias against the elderly concerning their potential for growth and change. Schaffer does not minimize the pain of aging. In fact, she deepens our appreciation for the ways in which physical, cognitive, and emotional losses of later life impact the self. What is remarkable is her ability to acknowledge the reality of her patients' experience while also helping them to know themselves better and find ways to grow. Her clinical illustrations expose the false dichotomy between supportive therapy and deep work, reflecting a humanity that is inspiring. Schaffer's voice has the potential to empower the therapist of aging patients who encounters their plight with a sense of helplessness and despair."

– **Martin Stephen Frommer, PhD,** Faculty, Stephen Mitchell Relational Study Center; Associate Editor, *Psychoanalytic Dialogues*

Blooming in December: Psychodynamic Psychotherapy with Older Adults

Amy Schaffer

Routledge
Taylor & Francis Group

LONDON AND NEW YORK

First published 2021
by Routledge
2 Park Square, Milton Park, Abingdon, Oxon OX14 4RN

and by Routledge
52 Vanderbilt Avenue, New York, NY 10017

Routledge is an imprint of the Taylor & Francis Group, an informa business

British Library Cataloguing-in-Publication Data
A catalogue record for this book is available from the British Library

Library of Congress Cataloging-in-Publication Data
Names: Schaffer, Amy, 1942– author.
Title: Blooming in December : psychodynamic psychotherapy with older adults / Amy Schaffer.
Description: Milton Park, Abingdon, Oxon ; New York, NY : Routledge, 2021. | Series: Psychoanalysis in a new key book series | Includes bibliographical references and index.
Identifiers: LCCN 2020048687 (print) | LCCN 2020048688 (ebook) | ISBN 9780367756437 (hardback) | ISBN 9780367756444 (paperback) | ISBN 9781003163343 (ebook)
Subjects: LCSH: Psychodynamic psychotherapy. | Older people—Psychology.
Classification: LCC RC489.P72 S33 2021 (print) | LCC RC489.P72 (ebook) | DDC 616.89/140846—dc23
LC record available at https://lccn.loc.gov/2020048687
LC ebook record available at https://lccn.loc.gov/2020048688

ISBN: 978-0-367-75643-7 (hbk)
ISBN: 978-0-367-75644-4 (pbk)
ISBN: 978-1-003-16334-3 (ebk)

Typeset in Times New Roman
by Apex CoVantage, LLC

Contents

Acknowledgments

Above all, I thank the patients whose work and growth in psychotherapy inspired this book. I am particularly indebted to those who allowed me to use material from their treatments in the clinical illustrations. I am deeply appreciative of the professional friends and colleagues, too numerous to mention here, who have contributed to my thinking about this topic and who have provided unfailing support. I thank Donnel Stern for his encouragement and guidance and Martin Frommer for his priceless feedback and nourishing dialogue. Words are insufficient to express my gratitude to Dominick Grundy for more than can be put on paper.

Chapter 1

Introduction

To work as a psychotherapist with older adults is to live with the painful reality of how little you can do. You cannot relieve arthritic pain or the agony of losing a spouse. You cannot cure cancer or fend off death. You cannot undo the wrong turns that your patient has taken earlier in life and now deeply regrets. And you cannot erase wrinkles. Yet, if you can tolerate these limitations, the work with this age group can be highly effective. It not only relieves suffering, but it can also lead to significant growth. And it can bring fulfillment and meaning to both patient and therapist.

Life's brevity, as Freud (1916) wrote in his poignant essay on transience, can make it all the sweeter. Older adults are all too aware of the fleeting nature of existence. And for many, the later years are indeed a time to treasure what life offers. For countless others, however, older age brings true distress. It brings depression, bitterness, feelings of failure, self-loathing, and shame. How do psychodynamic clinicians help suffering elders? An examination of the psychoanalytic literature provides little in the way of answers.

I have long wondered why psychoanalysts pay such scant attention to the treatment of the old. My interest in this population stems from an early experience running a group psychotherapy service for older adults. The psychiatrist head of the agency providing this service was open about his negative countertransference toward the aged. He was pessimistic about what therapy could offer these patients and expressed grateful surprise when the groups I led seemed to work. I loved these groups. I was a psychodramatically trained group therapist then, not yet trained in psychoanalysis. At the time I had led groups in several settings: two psychiatric hospitals, a residential camp for children with special needs, an institute treating young adults, and a service for creative artists. Of these many groups, those with the older adults stood out for the depth of connection of its members, their generosity toward each other, their willingness to reveal their vulnerabilities, their resilience and courage in the face of harsh life circumstances, and – particularly gratifying to a beginning therapist – how much benefit they seemed to gain from their groups. I learned from these groups and found them rewarding, inspiring.

Because I was vocal about my enthusiasm for this population, I have over the years received many referrals of older adults – including some from fellow therapists who referred their parents. At first, these patients were twice my age; now they are age-mates. Throughout, I have been mystified by the lack of interest by my colleagues in this group of potential patients.

Psychoanalytic writing on the aged, what there is of it, is extremely interesting. However, this literature is disturbingly sparse – especially so in proportion to the size of the population that can benefit from this treatment. Recently, attention is being paid to this lack of attention. McWilliams (2017), for example, described the neglect of later life in the first edition of the *Psychodynamic Diagnostic Manual* – ruefully noting the advanced ages of many involved in its creation and concluding: "We were a study in denial" (p. 51). Plotkin (2014) subtitled his urgent statement of the need for more focus on this area, "It's about time." Schachter et al. (2014) actually counted the number of papers on this topic to document their scarcity. And Junkers (2006) commented, "many analysts have a strange aversion to working clinically with elderly people" (p. xiii). Writers have begun to examine the prejudices responsible for this inattention (e.g., Wagner, 2005). And a small (so far) group of voices have begun to call for the work necessary to redress this imbalance, to examine the psychological needs of a significant and growing segment of our population. I join this chorus of voices and hope that others will as well. Let us embrace a quest to study how we can best serve people in their later years.

Is psychotherapy of older adults different from that of the young?

One might counter these voices, asking if there is really a need to further develop our theory about treatment at this stage of life. Doesn't existing psychodynamic theory adequately inform our work with these patients?

The answer is no. Of course, older adults are prey to the same difficulties as younger adults and, of course, existing psychodynamic theory is applicable to their treatment. But this theory while necessary is insufficient. Older patients face, and present to their therapists, unique issues and complexities. To offer just one example (many more will be discussed in the chapters ahead): a major thrust of our work with younger individuals is geared to fostering the development of, and removing the obstacles to, a sense of autonomy and agency. We want our patients to be captains of their ships. How then does one work with an 80-year-old who has achieved and prizes his autonomy and whose challenge now, in the face of physical infirmity, is to retain his sense of self and equanimity while experiencing ever-increasing dependence?

One's advanced years entail emotional challenges specific to this phase of life. The body changes in ways one cannot control and sphincters that used to work reliably no longer do. Social and familial roles are transformed. Indignities are many (Lax, 2008). Death looms and death anxiety can no longer be evaded. Losses pile up. Autonomy is diminished. Whatever was provided by the belief that one will have a future is no longer provided. And existential and spiritual questions surge to the surface. What has this all been about? Does my life have meaning? Who am I? Tested in this way, many people find their long-buried traumas and timeworn relational conflicts reemerging. Old defenses, which were once "good enough," no longer suffice. Issues that were worked through well enough in the past arise to be worked though again. Significant psychological effort is often required to meet these challenges. This effort can make the difference between a late life of fulfillment or of despair. And this effort is often fruitfully made within the context of a therapeutic relationship. But therapists of patients in this age group often work alone, grappling with emotions and questions in the absence of the grounding which a more complete literature, which a more complete dialogue between professionals, could provide.

With advances in our field – the expansion of our clinical repertoire, the movement of our theory from its emphasis on drives to one on relationship, our greater understanding of multiple modes of therapeutic action, and evidence of the neuroplasticity of the brain extending throughout the life span (Siegel, 2020) – we now have new and better conceptual tools for engaging in this work. My goal here will be to examine the psychological tasks of older age and the ways that the clinician can engage the older patient in work of depth and meaning, work promoting significant growth.

I send a cry to my fellow psychotherapists. Let us recognize that the population of older adults is increasing rapidly, that their mental health needs will be great. Let us study the later years as life spans lengthen. And let us rise to the occasion. It is incumbent upon us to learn more about how to help older people. In this work, I will examine what I have learned about the developmental crises and needs of older patients as well as the challenges they present to the clinician. I hope that in this goal I will be joined by many others.

I now turn to the factors that have contributed to the psychoanalytic world's striking lapse in attending to the treatment of older adults. Readers who would prefer to move directly to discussion of clinical work with this population may wish to skip this section and proceed to Chapter 2.

How is it that a field devoted to the psychological welfare of others has managed to keep its gaze from the needs of such a large sector of our human community? How is it that psychodynamic clinicians, individuals who constantly engage in self-analytic processes directed toward understanding their unconscious biases, have failed to recognize and grapple with *this* bias? The cumulative effect of numerous dynamics explains this glaring omission. It is imperative we face the multiple forces responsible for our lapse so that we can overcome them. I will begin with issues encountered by individual clinical practitioners which may lead to avoiding work with older patients. As significant as these may be, their effect is magnified by institutional hindrances stemming from the field of psychoanalysis. Our discipline, for all the richness and depth it offers, has been beset by biases that interfered with developing a solid foundation for treatment in the later stages of adulthood. I will, therefore, examine these institutional biases as well.

Challenges to the individual clinician in treating older patients

Psychodynamic treatment of the older patient can be extremely rewarding to the therapist but that is hardly the full story. It can also be excruciating. Some of the avoidance of this work stems from the difficulties it presents to the clinician. All of these have been made worse by the inadequacy of our theory and literature. Misery in the countertransference is not restricted to work with the old. We treat people with borderline personality disorder, we treat traumatized survivors of physical and sexual assault, and we treat addicts. We know that we will endure painful affects as we work with these populations. Gartner (2014), for example, summarizes his affective life working with sexually abused men, "However you look at it, it hurts" (p. 614). In the grip of the interpersonal field with these patients, we hurt. Fortunately, in these treatments our theory contains us. It helps us make sense of our experiences and puts words to them. Shared suffering is bearable suffering (Berzoff, 2019). This is true for our patients, and it is true for us. As the literature on working with elder patients grows and provides similar assistance to the therapist, I hope the challenges I describe below will become easier for therapists to bear.

Painful countertransference and assaults to grandiosity

The psychotherapist of the older patient must confront aging and death and must renounce the luxury of postponing this reckoning. To help these patients with their feelings and fears, we must face them ourselves. But, as Schramm (2018) comments, the elderly are sometimes (although not always) less frightened of death than are the professionals helping them. Humans are remarkably adroit at avoiding the knowledge that they will die (Becker, 1973). And in this respect, analysts are all too human. Too few create the professional wills which would ensure assistance to patients should the therapist be incapacitated. A long history of botched handling of therapist illness or death attests to this (Masur, 2018; O'Neil, 2013). Analysts such as Feinsilver (1998) and Gingold (2018), who faced terminal diagnoses and wrote about their thoughtful attempts to handle their practices therapeutically, are rare. I know of therapists who, denying their terminal illnesses, failed to inform their patients or to make provisions for their being informed – leaving these patients to learn of their therapists' deaths from a doorman or an obituary. I know of therapists who, unable or refusing to recognize their own dementia, insisted that their patients continue with them, interpreting their desires to leave therapy as resistance. Similar denial has manifested itself in cases where patients' expressions of reasonable fears about their infirm elderly therapists' possible deaths were interpreted as unconscious wishes to kill the therapist (Slochower, 2019). Psychoanalysts, like other mortals, avoid facing the realities of death and decline – even when the failure to do so harms others. Working as a therapist with patients in later life pierces this denial. Is it any wonder that members of our profession dodge such encounters?

Working with the aged also cracks into the analyst's comfortable and unacknowledged grandiosity. Under the sway of "Olympic delusions"

(Pinsky, 2017), we may unconsciously believe that we can defeat death. To work with the aged, we must face that despite our ministrations, patients die; that we, too, will die. Cooper (2016) reminds analysts of their need to continually rework the depressive position, pointing out that we have difficulty accepting our limits. In addition, it is not merely personal grandiosity which must be overcome but also psychoanalysts' idealization of psychoanalysis itself. As Gabbard (2017) observes, psychoanalysts may join their analysands in a shared unconscious fantasy of "triumph over death." To work with patients in late life is to tolerate the pain of relinquishing this illusion. This pain adds to the other aches that attend this work, aches further described in Chapter 4 on transference and countertransference.

Altered gratification from results

Psychoanalysts pride themselves on working for deep change. Not for us simple symptom relief. We want to make an internal transformation. We may name what we're after "structural change" or "modification of implicit memory systems" or "alteration of relational patterns" or "making the unconscious conscious" or "standing in the spaces." Whatever our terminology or psychoanalytic orientation, we are trying to influence our patients' inner life.

And yet, although these are our stated goals, it is striking that almost every case report in the literature describes external change as evidence of success. Our patients find mates, or blossom in their careers, or become better parents, or create art. These external gains, I believe, are described not merely because they demonstrate accomplishment but also because they are deeply gratifying to the therapist. And they should be. We work hard and long and experience joy when patients' external lives change for the better. Is this a pleasure one is denied in treating the aged? Not necessarily. In many cases, an older patient's external gains are highly gratifying to observe: a patient in late adulthood has his/her work shown in a gallery for the first time, makes a new friend, enjoys rather than quakes at a dinner party, confronts a financial consultant, accepts a long denied sexual orientation and has the courage to come out, or is finally able to feel and express loving feelings to a grandchild. But it is not uncommon for older patients to suffer a significant worsening of life's circumstances during treatment: a progressive disease progresses, a spouse's cognition deteriorates, impaired mobility (or vision or hearing) restricts or eliminates favorite activities, joints ache, siblings and childhood friends die, etc. Life narrows. Denied the pleasures of observing a patient's fuller external life, analysts must then be content with the satisfactions that come with recognition of internal change. Can a therapist be satisfied when the fruit of her therapeutic endeavors consists merely of decreased self-loathing, a more integrated and robust sense of self, a more cohesive and nuanced life narrative, an enhanced capacity for intimacy, greater peace of mind and an acceptance of an imperfect life well lived? And how does she value her work when despite these internal changes a patient's external life gets worse?

Ageism and unconscious normative processes

"Unlike all the bigotries now recognized as evil (among them sexism, racism and homophobia), 'ageism' has yet to become an everyday pejorative," writes Gullette (2017, p. 1). We live in a youth-obsessed society in which widespread biases devalue the old but remain relatively unrecognized. Psychoanalysis has had a poor track record for recognizing the psychic effects of social prejudice and the way these play themselves out in the treatment room. Fortunately, this has begun to change. There is now, for example, a significant and growing literature on the way race, class, and homophobia affect psyche and treatment. A similar effort must be made with respect to old age.

Ageism is one example of what Layton (2006) terms "normative unconscious processes." How do normative unconscious processes work? Layton summarizes the work of feminist theorists who have identified societal norms which idealize a form of middle-class masculinity in which autonomy is prized and dependency, human vulnerability, is devalued. Under the sway of these norms, people tend to split the wholeness of human experience into polarities and to project the undesirable parts of these experiences into others. In other words, rather than letting themselves experience the full range of human emotion, people will take an internal stance: "I am autonomous and strong; you are dependent and weak." These idealizations and projections play a big part in societal perceptions of categories, such as race, gender, class, and sexual orientation. Members of "othered" social groups are perceived as possessing disavowed, undesirable traits and as devoid of the more prized traits. Normative unconscious processes in this way perpetuate stereotypes which provide rationalizations for discrimination. Certain groups (e.g., blacks, women, and gays) are seen as possessing the less desirable, "bad" qualities (disowned by more privileged members of society) and hence as inferior.

How do normative unconscious processes affect our perceptions of the elderly? In a society that prizes autonomy, in a society that devalues and disowns human vulnerability, the manifestly vulnerable aged become the targets of projections. The non-old manage to avoid seeing their own vulnerabilities and they see the old as vulnerable, dependent, incapable, weak, and feminine. Of course, the non-old should more accurately be termed the not-yet-old. In discriminating against the aged, they/we are disowning not only vulnerable selves of the present but also feared selves of the future.

Psychotherapists are not exempt from normative unconscious processes including ageism. Out of our unconscious desires to disavow our own vulnerabilities, we may see the aged as more vulnerable than they are, as possessed of fewer strengths. Because these processes are unconscious, we remain unaware of them. What is more, as practitioners in one of the rare fields relatively untouched by this form of discrimination – we routinely continue to practice at ages where others would be unemployable – we have the luxury of blinding ourselves to the ageism in which we are immersed. The form this prejudice often takes is an underestimation of the capacities of older people. A common complaint among the aged is being talked to as if mentally deficient. And Freud's (1905) famous observation that people above the age of 50 are unlikely to change gave the stamp of authority to what is merely a prejudicial belief, that older people cannot benefit from psychoanalytic treatment, that they are incapable of psychic growth, and that they are unworthy of an analyst's time and effort.

Because so many in our field share these beliefs, let me take a moment to discredit this position. Are older adults too rigid to change? Hardly. Since the rigors of older age disrupt long-standing ways of being, older adults are often in a state of flux, with the potential either for breakdown or for reintegration at a higher level of functioning. Are older people too removed from their early lives to access memories of childhood experiences? No. Memory retrieval is not linear. Many elders report a resurgence of childhood memories. In addition, in the same way that a madeleine brought forth a host of memories for Proust, some of the sensory experiences of older age, sensations not felt since youth, provide a channel back to early memories. Finally, older people can be highly motivated to change. As Samuel Johnson put it, "When a man knows he is to be hanged in a fortnight, it concentrates his mind wonderfully." In other words, when an adult's denial of death is pierced, it creates an intensity that may actually speed up the therapy process. As Byock (2016) states, "Throughout life, crises that threaten the integrity of the person . . . offer the most opportunity for personal growth" (p. 286). Looming mortality is one of those crises. The powerful experience of facing one's mortality can catalyze growth.

Wrong turns: psychoanalytic history and the treatment of older patients

Sadly, psychoanalytic institutions themselves have fallen prey to our society's ageism and have enacted ageist policies. Plotkin (2019) has described in detail the obstacles he met in trying to use a septuagenarian patient, one eminently suitable for psychoanalytic work, as a control case. Turned down by his committee, he states, he received the permission he needed only by writing (in his words) "a shaming letter" to them, accusing them of falling short of psychoanalytic ideals in their display of prejudice. Eventually, they relented. But one wonders how many less assertive candidates simply gave up. The message was clear: psychoanalysis of older patients was unacceptable. Wagner (2005) similarly reports her institute's initial rejection of an octogenarian as a control case. "Although no one would deny the elderly supportive psychotherapy," she notes, "the possibility of psychoanalytic therapy still raises more eyebrows than genuine conviction" (p. 78). And Yu (2019) recounts receiving a phone call from an 83-year-old woman, eager to begin therapy, who had been turned down successively by numerous therapists who told her she was ineligible for psychoanalytic therapy because of her age. How many older adults have been deprived of beneficial treatment because of this prejudice? The damage we have done to potential patients as a result is disturbing to think about.

Psychoanalysts are trained to search for genetic roots: We look for the antecedents of individuals' "problems of living" in their histories. Our profession, however, has had difficulty in recognizing the way its own history has influenced, and at times compromised, its theory and practice. I have come to believe that three related aspects of psychoanalytic history have impeded our field's ability to conceptualize and value the treatment of older patients: (1) the profound effects of the Holocaust on the early psychoanalysts; (2) the tensions and competitions in the field, which resulted in a sharp delineation between psychoanalysis and (much lower status) psychotherapy; and (3) the failure of the field to adequately conceptualize phenomena, such as late-onset trauma, attachment, loss, and death anxiety.

Twentieth-century history and psychoanalytic rigidity

Prince (2009) and Kuriloff (2014) have performed illuminating analyses of the effects of the Holocaust on American psychoanalysis. The originators of psychoanalysis in this country were predominantly Europeans who, in varying ways, suffered extremes of loss, helplessness, lack of safety, and dislocation during the Holocaust. In short, many of our pioneers were both brilliant and traumatized. Their bravery, resilience, and initiative in developing the field of psychoanalysis in this context are truly admirable and a great gift to those who followed. But the degree of trauma they suffered was not without consequence.

Among the sequelae of the trauma of the Holocaust was a stance which severely curtailed effective therapeutic work with the aged. That is, both out of a need to hold fast to the old (i.e., the world they had lost, the leader they had lost) and to be acceptable to and gain status in the new (i.e., the country to which they had immigrated), prominent psychoanalysts adopted a stance of theoretical rigidity.

Unfortunately, mid-century American-born psychoanalysts joined their immigrant colleagues in this inflexibility. Richards (2016), who has studied the leftist affiliations of these analysts, speculates that they were influenced by the authoritarianism which characterized socialist organizations, such as the American Communist Party and the USSR. In any case, whatever the contribution of these historical forces, mid-20th-century psychoanalysis was characterized by a high degree of rigidity with respect to training procedures, theory, and prescribed methods of practice.

Among the detrimental features of a too-rigid traditional analysis were an overreliance on oedipal dynamics as the etiology of pathology, the definition of psychoanalysis by its frame (at least four times/week on the couch) rather than by the nature of the work, adherence to a stringent standard of anonymity, neutrality and abstinence on the part of the analyst, lack of recognition that influence in the therapeutic dyad goes two ways, and an overarching belief in interpretation of the transference as the main ingredient of therapeutic action. Ironically, in maintaining such an austere, inflexible model of psychoanalysis, these leaders in the field were depart-ing from the example set by Freud. On occasion, Freud gave his patients food, vacationed with them, and wrote affectionate letters (Lipton, 1977). I have sometimes wondered if he would have had trouble graduating from a psychoanalytic institute in postwar America!

One negative consequence of this traditional psychoanalytic stringency is described by Straker (2013), who for decades has led discussion groups for psychoanalytically trained professionals who treat the terminally ill. He has found a common and uncomfortable countertransference among these clinicians stemming from the fact that to accommodate the medical needs of their patients, they must modify the traditional psychoanalytic frame. These worthy clinicians, dedicated to helping patients *in extremis*, feel guilty. Although they know that deviations from the basic model of psychoanalysis are necessary and in the best interest of the patient, they feel bad at straying from the fold, at abandoning the technique they have been taught. In other words, doing good therapy makes them guilty. The stringency of traditional psychoanalysis has produced harsh psychoana-lytic superegos!

The inferior status of psychodynamic psychotherapy

Aron and Starr (2013) add to the picture of the forces militating to uphold and maintain this rigid definition of psychoanalysis in their description of decades-long bruising battles over the boundary between psychoanaly-sis and psychodynamic psychotherapy. To summarize their complex and cogent argument briefly: In love with the vision of themselves as pos-sessors of the scientific knowledge of how to cure, psychoanalysts made a sharp distinction between "curing" and "caring," relegating caring to inferior status. There was a misogynistic cast to this distinction, since males were the ones with the scientific knowledge who cured and females were the ones who provided care. The requirement of a medical degree for psychoanalysts (a requirement opposed by Freud) added to the misogyny, since few women were admitted to medical schools. The medical require-ment also created a hierarchy in which mental health professionals with other degrees could not receive psychoanalytic training and had lower sta-tus. (Psychologists eventually took legal action in order to gain access to the field.)

Good treatment of older patients requires flexibility, departures from traditional ways of working. Frames must be modified to allow for the necessity of inconsistent frequency, of contact with family members, of a therapist helping her patient up the stairs or paying a hospital visit. Abstinence, the limiting of intervention to interpretation, and the failure to recognize mutual influence are all detrimental in work with older patients. When psychoanalytic treatment was defined rigidly, when legitimacy was defined by adherence to old norms rather than by the depth of the work, effective therapy of older adults looked unacceptable, "un-psychoanalytic." It was deemed "supportive therapy" and given low status.

This means that in the past psychoanalysts treating older adults could not give patients what was needed if they wanted to conform to the standards psychoanalysts had created for themselves. In addition, unless practitioners managed somehow to make their treatments of older patients conform to traditional standards, their clinical reports were unpublishable in psychoanalytic journals. That was certainly sufficient reason to avoid (or at least to avoid writing about) this work. "Many more psychoanalysts are treating older people than has been reported," writes Yu (2007, p. 443). The failure to incorporate their work into what is deemed acceptable psychodynamic practice has delayed our field's development of expertise with this population.

Traditional psychoanalytic practice had rationales for its inelasticity. Many of the characteristics of traditional technique served, it was believed, to create the necessary environment conducive to deep psychic change. Strachey (1934), in his highly influential paper on therapeutic action, proposed that this technique creates "the point of urgency" for patients. That is, it brings into the transference the emotional intensity that is requisite for therapeutic effectiveness, rendering transference interpretations powerfully mutative. In contrast with this view, I have found these prerequisites to creating "urgency" are unnecessary with patients of all ages – but particularly with the old. As I noted earlier, quoting Samuel Johnson, the proximity of death concentrates the mind wonderfully. Older patients with or without a traditional psychoanalytic frame can have intense psychotherapeutic experiences and can dig very deep indeed.

Blind spots

The denied or dissociated trauma of psychoanalytic pioneers may also be responsible for a weakness in our field which has always puzzled me. That is, the trauma and loss our forebears suffered may explain in part the difficulties psychoanalysis long had in theorizing a trio of significant parts of human experience: trauma, loss and mourning, and the facing of death. Whatever the origin of these lapses, each of these areas, of profound relevance to the psychotherapy of the elderly, was either neglected or misconceived (or both) for much of psychoanalytic history. And these delays in psychoanalytic understanding left practitioners ill-equipped to meet the needs of an older population.

Trauma

That psychoanalysis had some mishaps along its way to developing an understanding of trauma is now widely accepted by psychoanalysts. Freud's abandonment of the seduction hypothesis moved the field into an unfortunate focus on fantasy as the etiology of pathology, obliterating recognition of the reality of sexual trauma and its aftermath (Davies & Frawley, 1994). In addition, analytic theory, which firmly planted the origin of psychopathology in childhood experience, failed to recognize the existence and significance of trauma occurring later. "It is as if psychoanalytic theory itself denies or dissociates the possibilities of reactions to late-onset trauma," observed Boulanger (2002, p. 19). The extent of our field's blindness to post-childhood trauma can be seen in the reports by concentration camp survivors that their analysts discouraged their discussing their lives in the camps and instead focused on intrapsychic conflicts stemming from early childhood (Kuriloff, 2014). One of the unfortunate effects of this lapse may be the way it hindered our understanding and treatment of older patients. As I will discuss further in Chapter 3, the treatment of older adults requires an understanding of late-onset trauma. A patient falls, breaks a hip, and lies in pain on her kitchen floor for 3 days until help arrives. Another has a heart attack on a New York City subway and fears for her belongings and her life. A third has a stroke and is suddenly incontinent and unable to walk. To comprehend the direct impact of these events (as well as the way they revive earlier experiences of suffering) and to help patients deal with them requires an understanding of trauma which early psychoanalysis eschewed.

Attachment/loss/mourning

Psychoanalytic theorists were slow to recognize the importance and relevance of attachment theory (Holmes, 1993). One chilling example of the failure to recognize the power of attachment is reported by Kuriloff (2014): the case of a boy who lost his mother in the Holocaust. Strikingly, this child's difficulties were *not* identified as stemming from this loss. Instead, intrapsychic conflict was the focus, and the child was deemed to be too dependent on his mother. Older adults often suffer massive losses. It would not be unusual for an older patient to lose within 1 year a spouse, a sibling, and several childhood friends. The psychological challenges of old age include finding ways to navigate these losses. A therapist's recognition and understanding of the power of attachment and loss are, therefore, crucial.

Help with mourning is an important part of the therapist's work and, again, a part that was ill-served by earlier psychoanalytic theory. For dependent on an "energic" model of mental functioning, analysts viewed successful mourning as requiring the eventual removal of libidinal energy from the one who is lost. In this way, the energy would be free to be invested in (cathected to) someone else. As I will discuss further in Chapter 7, we now know that this view is mistaken, that ties to those loved and lost must be transformed, not dissolved.

Facing death and death anxiety

Freud believed that death could not be represented in the unconscious. His ideas, in Yalom's words (1980), "begat a cult of death denial in generations of therapist" (p. 66). Hoffman (1998), reviewing the literature of these generations, concluded: "relatively little attention has been paid to the process by which the individual anticipates, reacts to and comes to terms with his or her own death" (p. 31). And Piven (2003) observed that while over the years brilliant articles had been written on the subject, they had been almost uniformly ignored.

It's not as if patients never expressed their fears of death. But these were most often conceived of as covers for other deeper anxieties, such as the fear of castration. (To interpret an 85-year-old's death terror as a derivative of castration anxiety certainly entailed mental gymnastics!) Any treatment may require the exploration of the meaning of death. But in the treatment of the elderly, this work is paramount. In fact, to avoid this topic is to do a grave disservice (pun intended). It is important to explore patients' representations, fantasies and ideas about death, their early experiences with death, the models of dying provided by their parents, and the emotional valences they bring to the knowledge that they will die.

In addition, it is important to do this in the context of a certain kind of relatedness. Unfortunately, the austerity of the therapist required in the earlier versions of psychoanalysis precluded providing what was needed. For, in Frommer's (2016) words, "Mortality seeks relationality" (p. 373). As psychoanalysis has shifted to the relational, we are no longer forbidden to offer what the older patient facing death needs from us: an engagement in which two vulnerable humans ponder their mortality.

Qualifications and limitations

I will not be writing about helping those whose deaths are imminent, who are in the final portion of the final stage. This is a specialized area, one in which I am neither trained nor experienced. Fortunately, there are ways to receive this training, such as that provided in preparation for hospice work or by teachers of the Buddhist tradition of Contemplative Care. I look forward to the day when this body of knowledge is integrated with our psychodynamic understandings, so that we can provide better care to those in their final days.

Throughout my career, I have always had a few older adults in my practice. The populations of older adults I have treated and will be using as case examples do not constitute a representative sample of older adults in this country. Almost all were referred to me by someone who knew me. Some were referred by colleagues, some by former patients, and some by friends. They have all lived in the greater metropolitan New York City area. Most of them, although by no means all, have been white. Most of them, although by no means all, have been born in this country but have varying ethnic and religious backgrounds. More have been women than have been men. I have always used a sliding-scale fee structure and their economic situations have varied widely. Although many had financial worries, none have been homeless or lacked the basic necessities of life. None have lived in assisted living facilities or in nursing homes. None were facing, to their knowledge, imminent death. All have at the beginning of their treatments been able to come to see me in my office. A few, eventually too disabled to travel to me, have had their sessions by phone. On a few occasions, I have paid hospital or home visits but not often.

I believe that much of what I will be talking about in this book will be generalizable to older adults in different circumstances. And I look forward to the contributions of others in finding ways to do meaningful psychodynamic work with older adults of many backgrounds and in many settings.

To protect confidentiality, in providing clinical illustrations, I have altered details of my patients' lives. Occasionally I have blended information from more than one patient to create a composite.

I move now into what my practice of psychodynamic psychotherapy with older adults has taught me and the way I have come to conceptualize this work. In Chapter 2, I will discuss the developmental tasks from earlier years which reemerge in older age and revive earlier relational conflicts and trauma. Chapter 3 will focus on trauma, both that precipitated by the depredations of older age and that revived from childhood. In Chapter 4, I will explore the transference/countertransference configurations frequently met in work with older adults and the requirement that therapists study their own biases. The focus in Chapter 5 will be on the way the modification and enrichment of the life narrative in later years strengthen the sense of self. Chapter 6 will center on existential issues: death as a felt experience, the search for meaning and the recognition of one's lack of omnipotence. In Chapter 7, I will discuss endings and mourning.

References

Aron, L., & Starr, K. (2013). *A psychotherapy for the people: Toward a progressive psychoanalysis*. Routledge.

Becker, E. (1973). *The denial of death*. The Free Press.

Berzoff, J. (2019). Being still: Sitting with suffering in long-term relational practice. In S. A. Lord (Ed.), *Reflections on long-term relational psychotherapy and psychoanalysis: Relational analysis interminable* (pp. 119–131). Routledge.

Boulanger, G. (2002). The cost of survival: Psychoanalysis and adult onset trauma. *Contemporary Psychoanalysis, 38*(1), 17–44.

Byock, I. (2016). Imagining people well. In K. P. Ellison & M. Weingast (Eds.), *Awake at the bedside: Contemplative teachings on palliative and end-of-life care* (pp. 281–297). Wisdom Publications.

Cooper, S. H. (2016). *The analyst's experience of the depressive position: The melancholic errand of psychoanalysis*. Routledge.

Davies, J. M., & Frawley, M. G. (1994). *Treating the adult survivor of childhood sexual abuse: A psychoanalytic perspective*. Basic Books.

Feinsilver, D. B. (1998). The therapist as a person facing death: The hardest of external realities and therapeutic action. *International Journal of Psycho-Analysis, 79*, 1131–1150.

Freud, S. (1905). On psychotherapy. In J. Strachey (Ed. & Trans.), *The standard edition of the complete psychological works of Sigmund Freud* (Vol. 7, pp. 265–268). Hogarth Press.

Freud, S. (1916). On transience. In J. Strachey (Ed & Trans.), *The standard edition of the complete psychological works of Sigmund Freud* (Vol. 14, pp. 303–307). Hogarth Press.

Frommer, M. (2016). Death is nothing at all: On contemplating non-existence. A relational psychoanalytic engagement of the fear of death. *Psychoanalytic Dialogues, 26*(4), 373–390.

Gabbard, G. O. (2017). Sexual boundary violations in psychoanalysis: A 30-year retrospective. *Psychoanalytic Psychology, 34*(2), 151–156.

Gartner, R. B. (2014). Trauma and countertrauma, resilience and counterresilience. *Contemporary Psychoanalysis, 50*(4), 609–626.

Gingold, H. (2018). On telling your patients you are going to die: An analytic odyssey. *NYS Psychologist, 30*(1), 59–65.

Gullette, M. M. (2017). *Ending ageism, or how not to shoot old people*. Rutgers University Press.

Hoffman, I. Z. (1998). *Ritual and spontaneity in the analytic process: A dialectical-constructivist view*. Analytic Press.

Holmes, J. (1993). *John Bowlby and attachment theory*. Routledge.

Junkers, G. (2006). *Is it too late? Key papers on psychoanalysis and aging*. Karnak.

Kuriloff, E. A. (2014). *Contemporary psychoanalysis and the legacy of the Third Reich*. Routledge.

Lax, R. F. (2008). Becoming really old: The indignities. *Psychoanalytic Quarterly, 77*(3), 835–857.

Layton, L. (2006). Racial identities, racial enactments and normative unconscious processes. *The Psychoanalytic Quarterly, 75*(1), 237–269.

Lipton, S. D. (1977). The advantages of Freud's technique as shown in his analysis of the rat man. *International Journal of Psycho-Analysis, 58*, 255–273.

Masur, C. (2018). Mortality and psychoanalysis: The analyst's defense against acknowledging mortality and the effect on clinical practice. In C. Masur (Ed.), *Flirting with death: Psychoanalysts consider mortality* (pp. 7–24). Routledge.

McWilliams, N. (2017). Psychoanalytic reflections on limitation: Aging, dying, generativity, and renewal. *Psychoanalytic Psychology, 34*(1), 50–57.

O'Neil, M. K. (2013). Now is the time for action: The professional will: An ethical responsibility of the analyst and the profession. In G. Junkers (Ed.), *The empty couch: The taboo of ageing and retirement in psychoanalysis* (pp. 150–160). Routledge.

Pinsky, E. (2017). *Death and fallibility in the analytic encounter: Mortal gifts*. Routledge.

Piven, J. S. (2003). Introduction. *The Psychoanalytic Review, 90*(4), 395–402.

Plotkin, D. A. (2014). Older adults and psychoanalytic treatment: It's about time. *Psychodynamic Psychiatry, 42*(1), 23–50.

Plotkin, D. A. (2019, February 9). *Aging: Another inconvenient truth*. Paper Chinese American Psychoanalytic Alliance Conference on Eastern and Western Views of Aging, New York, NY.

Prince, R. (2009). Psychoanalysis traumatized: The legacy of the holocaust. *American Journal of Psychoanalysis, 69*(3), 179–194.

Richards, A. D. (2016). The left and far left in American psychoanalysis: Psychoanalysis as a subversive discipline. *Contemporary Psychoanalysis, 52*(1), 111–129.

Schachter, J., Kächele, H., & Schachter, J. S. (2014). Psychotherapeutic/psychoanalytic treatment of the elderly. *Psychodynamic Psychiatry, 42*(1), 51–63.

Schramm, M. G. (2018). A death in the family: Report of a single session trauma group for nursing home residents and staff. *International Journal of Group Psychotherapy, 68*(3), 297–313.

Siegel, D. J. (2020). *The developing brain: How relationships and the brain interact to shape who we are* (3rd ed.). Guilford Press.

Slochower, J. (2019, February 25–March 2). *Trying not to look ahead*. Anne and Ramon Alonso Plenary Address. American Group Psychotherapy Association Annual Conference, Los Angeles, CA.

Strachey, J. (1934). On the nature of the therapeutic action of psychoanalysis. *International Journal of Psycho-Analysis, 15*, 127–159.

Straker, N. (Ed.). (2013). *Facing cancer and the fear of death: Psychoanalytic perspectives on treatment*. Rowman & Littlefield.

Wagner, J. J. (2005). Psychoanalytic bias against the elderly patient: Hiding our fears under developmental millstones. *Contemporary Psychoanalysis, 41*(1), 77–92.

Yalom, I. D. (1980). *Existential psychotherapy*. Basic Books.

Yu, M. (2007). Across generations, genders and cultures: A young Chinese-born woman treats an American-born nonagenarian Jewish man. *Contemporary psychoanalysis, 43*(3), 421–444.

Yu, M. (2019, February 9). *Old country, new country: Culture and countertransference*. Paper Presented at Chinese American Psychoanalytic Alliance Conference on Eastern and Western Views of Aging, New York, NY.

Chapter 2

Ghosts in later life

"I can't open my bedroom window," announced Sadie, a widow in her late 60s, to her therapy group. "What should I do? Should I ask my super to help? If I ask him, should I tip him? If I don't tip him enough, though, will he shun me afterwards? I guess I could wait until my son-in-law visits and ask him. But what if he starts thinking I'm a burdensome old lady? Maybe I should just get used to sleeping in an airless room."

I, the group leader, listened to Sadie and thought, "This is going to be an incredibly boring group." A stuck window seemed a less-than-riveting opening for a discussion of any depth. I was, therefore, surprised by the vibrant conversation that ensued. Group members described their own experiences and talked, at times with deep feeling, about what it was like to need help, about the humiliation that came with loss of self-sufficiency, the worry about the trustworthiness of the people you had to rely on, the shift in your self-concept when you felt incapable of doing things you used to be able to do, and the shattering moments when you realized that your spouse would never again be there to help.

This group took place over 40 years ago. At the time, I realized that Sadie's feelings about her stuck window and the potent responses of others to her situation were a clue to something I needed to understand. Sadie's window represented not merely a physical challenge but also an emotional one – a challenge all the group members seemed to understand and share. What happens in later life which would explain the impact of such a concrete event? What made Sadie's stuck window such compelling material for a group?

To answer that question, I begin by borrowing from the work of Erik Erikson (1984, 1998). Most early psychoanalytic theorists focused solely on the first years of life, but Erikson, with the collaboration of his wife Joan, devised a theory of human development which examined the entire life span as a progression through a series of eight stages during each of which the individual faces a critical task. Later the theory was amended to include a ninth stage in late life, one in which the challenges previously faced arise again and must be re-confronted. Without subscribing to the orderly progression of stages included in Erikson's theory, I will focus on the developmental tasks he identified – for these do indeed arise to rechallenge in later life. Sadie's dilemma and the discussion it sparked in her group, for example, can be seen as revolving around issues of trust and autonomy, conflicts from Erikson's first two stages.

I propose that these returning earlier challenges bring with them what I think of as "ghosts." That is, the return of the developmental tasks of one's earlier years often revives the relational conflicts and trauma of those times. Issues that have been laid to rest sufficiently for a degree of stability throughout adulthood may come roaring back to life. These reawakened conflicts and their accompanying ghosts may jeopardize equanimity and quality of life. For the sad fact is that the problematic experiences of one's early years often gain greater disruptive power later, as the hardships that accompany older age and the facing of the end of one's existence revive long-buried troubles. In older age, previously high-functioning people may enter into states of deadened despair, of rageful belligerence, or of inconsolable misery. When that happens, the combination of current and revived tribulations can stymie successful adaptation. The remedy to this situation often entails taking on long-quiescent problems from one's earlier life. Fortunately, the destabilization of this period also affords opportunity, for disintegration can lead to reintegration at a higher level. Psychotherapeutic help offered at this time may both reduce suffering and result in significant psychological growth.

I will continue later with these ideas and then conclude with an illustrative case. First, however, I return to the therapy groups with which I started, for these were where I had my first vivid lessons about the psychological tasks of older age.

In Chapter 1, I described my position as a therapy group leader in the '70s. During that period, for over 5 years, I ran two weekly groups of patients aged 60 and older. Most came because they were patients of my employer, a psychiatrist with a practice on New York City's Upper East Side; the groups were held on his premises. Others came through word of mouth or because they met me at open-to-the-public workshops in which I invited older adults to discuss themes related to aging. All members of the groups were roughly twice my age or older; most, although not all, were women. Relying on my psychodrama training, I often began these groups with simple warm-up and role-playing exercises. (For an introduction to these techniques, see Blatner, 1997; Leveton, 1977.) These inevitably led to deeply personal discussions in which group members shared their experiences, feelings, and quandaries. Laughter, tears, and intimate exchanges were frequent. I found the groups moving, funny and illuminating. I sometimes wondered who was getting more out of these groups, the group members or me.

From Sadie, I had learned about the way issues surrounding dependency and trust can reemerge in one's later years. I learned about a second set of issues when a retired corporate executive – let's call him Leon – started a group by venting the frustration he experienced when, upon volunteering to help at a local non-profit, he was given low-level clerical work to do. He had the skills to make the organization function more effectively, yet his managerial prowess remained both ignored and unused. "I showed them my resume," he stated sadly, "and they put me to work stuffing envelopes." Another group member jumped in quickly to commiserate. A former high school teacher, she had suffered a depression when retiring because nothing she now did gave her the respect from others and the self-respect that teaching had offered. The group joined in with an animated discussion of changed social roles, feelings of diminished competence and worth, and altered senses of identity.

Rose, recently widowed, started another meeting by talking about her conflict with her daughter. The daughter, seeing Rose's loneliness, wanted her to join a senior citizen center. How could a chat with a few elderly people she had just met replace the closeness she had had with her husband of 50 years, Rose sobbed? And, it felt awful, she told the group, after a lifetime in which she took good care of her daughter to now have her daughter trying (ineffectively!) to take care of her. The group members were empathic with Rose and shared how they were coping with their own experiences of loss and how painful it was that they could no longer be the givers but instead were the given to.

In another group, Jane addressed the widows who had been discussing the pain of widowhood, stating that she was embarrassed to tell them something. "While you are suffering so much from the loss of your husband," she told Rose, "I am miserable because I have too much of mine." The group questioned her and learned that her husband, a pharmacist, had just retired. From a schedule that had kept him out of their home 6 days a week from 8 a.m. to 6 p.m., he was now there full-time. She could not stand having him around, had recently pulled a mattress into a spare room and was sleeping on the floor. Painfully and with tears, several group members shared stories about their once relatively happy marriages going sour following changes due to a spouse's retirement, illness, cognitive decline, or depression. Intimacy had fled their lives.

Before leaving these groups of the 1970s, let me add something else I learned – not from a group meeting but from an evaluation form I gave to all group members for assessment purposes. Among the many questions on the form was one in which I listed several possible topics and asked group members to put a check mark next to any topic they would like us to focus on more. I remember only two items on the list, in both cases because the responses to them were unexpected. These were the '70s, the days when Kübler-Ross's (1969) ideas on death and dying were being widely disseminated, so I reasoned that group members might welcome an opportunity to talk about death. Not a single person had checked "death." (It was only years later that I realized that their responses might have reflected not so much an avoidance of the topic but rather an avoidance of talking about it with a group leader in her 30s!) A majority of group members had, however, checked "sex." In this way, I learned that sexual desire and interest persist in older age.

Development in later life

In one of the great and most often cited papers of our field, Loewald (1960) described the major goal of psychoanalysis. Our aim, he stated, is to help set development back in motion. It requires of the analyst, he added, love and respect for the individual and for the individual's development. If this is our task, how does it apply to the older patient? What represents successful development in older age? And how does the psychodynamic psychotherapist, with love and respect, foster this development?

In its original version Erikson's theory included the following eight stages: (1) basic trust vs. mistrust, (2) autonomy vs. shame or doubt, (3) initiative vs. guilt, (4) industry vs. inferiority, (5) identity vs. identity confusion, (6) intimacy vs. isolation, (7) generativity vs. stagnation, and

(8) ego integrity vs. despair and disgust. At each of these stages, the individual's critical task was to face the polarity Erikson named and to arrive at a solution weighted toward the more positive of the two poles. For example, in successful development, the infant would optimally develop a sufficient degree of trust, as opposed to mistrust, to serve as a foundation for dealing with the later developmental challenges. In the eighth stage, the individual's developmental task was to avoid despair, establish ego integrity, and in the process ascend to wisdom. This was, for decades, the analytic view of development in later life.

As the Eriksons aged, they recognized their theory's inadequacy, that older age presents hurdles they hadn't envisioned. Erik Erikson commented on his earlier understanding of the eighth stage, "the demand to develop Integrity and Wisdom in old age seems to be somewhat unfair, especially when made by middle-aged theorists – as, indeed, we then were" (1984, p. 159). And Joan Erikson (1998), in discussing the reemergence of old conflicts, emphasized the arduous nature of this reworking with her suggestion (made when she was 93!) that in their late-life iteration the stages should be renamed by reversing the order of the concepts. The developmental conflicts of the ninth stage are so taxing, she believed, that the negative concept should be named first. In other words, while the infant faces the conflict "basic trust vs. basic mistrust," the elder adult is met by "basic mistrust vs. trust."

I am generally suspicious of stage theories and I am not alone in this uneasiness. Increasingly, psychoanalysts have questioned the assumption of a linear progression which provides the foundation for any stage theory. They question whether the complex permutations of human development can be reasonably described as following a single trajectory (e.g., Wagner, 2005). Divorced from the framework of successive stages, however, the conflicts Erikson identified are conceptually useful. And the Eriksons were correct: They do return in older age.

The group experiences reported earlier provide evidence. Sadie's inability to open her window brought up a heightened sense of dependency and along with it mistrust of others and feelings of decreased autonomy. Leon's retirement required him to find new ways of feeling competence and of retaining his identity. Rose was dealing not only with loss of intimacy and grief but also with the blow to her generativity when her daughter wanted to take care of her. Jane found her capacity for intimacy overburdened and disintegrating following her husband's retirement. The assaults of aging required these people to find fresh solutions to old issues. As the Eriksons' revised theory predicted, they were reencountering earlier challenges. Group members, after perhaps decades of relative stability in managing conflicts over trust, autonomy, competence, identity, loving, and caring, had to find new resolutions.

Relational conflicts revived and the return of ghosts

Loewald (1960) described the desired result of therapy: "The ghosts of the unconscious are laid and led to rest as ancestors whose power is taken over and transformed into the newer intensity of present life" (p. 29). Unfortunately, many ghosts, laid to rest – or at least kept at bay – in one's earlier life, revive and haunt in older age. It is not merely the aging body and mind which make later life so difficult. Rather, this is when ghosts return, the ghosts of early relational difficulties and early trauma.

For an example, let us return to Sadie. Sadie faces a current, real-life predicament and a distasteful experience of dependency. Early relational experiences, however, will contribute to the affects, the experience of self and the experience of others she brings to this dilemma. If, for example, Sadie came from a family in which self-sufficiency was prized and those soliciting help were shamed, she might have an internalized relationship we could name "Seeker of Help/Disparager of the Seeker." If the awakening of this relational conflict leads her to persecute herself internally when she needs help, dealing with her stuck window will become very unpleasant indeed. On the other hand, if Sadie had an over-doting parent who met her every need before she even asked, sending the message that she was incapable of self-care and entitled to rescue, her internalized relational configuration might be named "Helpless Needy Little Girl/Undermining Rescuer." If that were the case, Sadie's need for help might evoke feelings of inadequacy and an expectation of being rescued. In either case, as her body aged, Sadie's increased need for physical assistance in older age would revive the ghosts of earlier years and would affect the way she experienced greater dependency.

A question may arise here. If Sadie has these internalized relational conflicts, why are they emerging only now, in her elder years? Why weren't they troubling her before? And the answer is that of course such issues would have arisen in her earlier life and have created conflict at times. In older age, however, these earlier issues might come flooding back with unprecedented power.

Why now?

Why do earlier issues erupt in later life with such urgency? There are a host of reasons. Many earlier developmental achievements are linked to the body's evolution from the helplessness of infancy to the flower of full adulthood. For example, the mastery of sphincter control and the ability to walk independently foster the development of autonomy. In older age, the physical capacities decline. The individual may be challenged, for example, to retain a sense of autonomy while suffering urinary incontinence and impaired mobility.

Relational conflicts may become manifest because older age requires a return to relational configurations not experienced since childhood. Needing help from the other, feeling physically weaker than the other, not being able to keep up with the other, and having difficulty learning new tasks that the other can easily master – these relational experiences, endemic to childhood, may bring back the feelings and relational patterns from those years.

In older age, familiar defenses may no longer be available. Someone, for example, with conflicts about autonomy might have been able to manage these anxieties with activities which evoked feelings of potency – say, stockpiling money, running marathons, or pursuing sexual conquest. In older age, these types of defenses no longer work. Greenberg (2016), writing about psychodynamic psychotherapy with older adults who are ill, notes that people who relied on manic defenses – with which they fended off humiliating feelings of vulnerability and dependency with illusions of power – may have particular difficulty when these defenses fail in older age.

In addition, in one's later years, new trauma can trigger old trauma. Physical illness, unrelenting pain, loss of attachment figures, and experiences rendering one helpless can revive the emotional memories of early traumatic ordeals. Self-states long sequestered by dissociation may emerge. In addition, facing the fragility of life and the knowledge one will die may evoke terror. Death may become a giant Rorschach onto which the horrors of past traumas are projected. I will be discussing this phenomenon at greater length in Chapter 3.

Growth in older age via psychotherapy

Are older adults, as Freud (1905) posited, too rigid to change? Are their relational patterns so encrusted, the origins of their conflicts so buried, and their psyches so beset by concrete considerations that growth is impossible? I believe not. The discovery by neurologists that neuroplasticity is not limited to the younger years, but persists throughout life, supports my view.

I do not want to be a Pollyanna here. Life can indeed be cruel to older people and not all endings are happy. Also, while many older adults are capable of growth spurts and increased self-realization, there may be numerous obstacles that prevent this positive outcome. An individual's physical condition, living situation, financial status, and social environment influence greatly the degree of difficulty in accomplishing the developmental tasks of older age. The gravity of these obstacles cannot be underestimated. In its earlier years, psychoanalysis was negligent in recognizing the impact of realities on patients' lives. Let us not make that mistake. The conditions under which elderly people in our society often live are appalling and hardly conducive to mental health, much less emotional growth. The ageism in our society, the isolation of our elders and their sequestration in barren environments, the lack of financial security, the torturous routes to decent medical care, and the lack of support they often face – all these can play a major role in making older age a time of misery. In addition, issues such as major illness, chronic pain, impaired mobility, cognitive deterioration, and successive losses of attachment figures exact their toll. Urgent bodily concerns, moreover, as Greenberg (2016) observes, can render thinking concrete. During periods where those prevail, psychotherapists can provide empathic attunement and meet attachment needs for security but must await the restoration of reflective function for deeper work. Psychotherapy is not magic – but for a significant number of older adults, it can make a huge difference.

Older adults often undergo a process both like and unlike "regression in the service of development" (Blos, 1968), the retreat to an earlier developmental level to foster maturational advancement. This concept has been applied to adolescents who seem to lose their maturity, to go "backwards," in order to mature. The travails of older age often do provoke a regression-like phenomenon in which the individual is plunged back into the conflicts and relational patterns of earlier years. To name this "regression" is to ignore the maturational achievement and strengths that the individual retains even during these times. An older adult may be reimmersed in struggles from early life but is accompanied there by a wealth of life experience and learning. As in "regression in the service of development," however, there is a dissolution of old ways of being which increases plasticity and provides the potential for fruitful, deep change.

Gerson (2018) addresses the profound psychological effect on an adult of the death of a parent. (I will return to a discussion of her work in Chapter 7.) This major life event, she notes, can induce an internal malleability allowing internalized object representations to be modified. Older age – during which the death of siblings, spouses, partners, friends, and, ultimately, the self must be faced – can, similarly, catalyze the psychic fluidity requisite for profound change. And thus, although the frame with older patients may look little like the traditional frame, the depth of the work, and the change achieved may be what traditional analytic technique aimed for. In working with elders, often a little goes a long way. Thus, while our older patients continue to suffer all the hardships and indignities of aging, they may also experience the joy of new and richer experiences.

Claire

Patients who return to therapy in later life often illustrate the extent to which early issues, issues that have previously reached "good enough" resolutions, spring back to life in older age. Such was the case with Claire.

Claire, a retired widow in her mid-70s, sought therapy because she was depressed, was fighting with her daughter-in-law and with friends, and saw no point in living. She had undertaken a full and very helpful analysis when she was in her 30s and 40s, she told me. (Her previous analyst, famous enough that I was somewhat intimidated at the idea of following in her footsteps, had died.) "I should have come to you sooner," she said. "Ever since I turned 70, I've been having dreams of houses in disrepair with pipes leaking and walls crumbling."

One day Claire arrived at my office following a medical appointment, saying: "He says I have a blocked carotid. He told me to stay away from animal fats, to stop eating butter. But I'm not going to listen to him. What nonsense! Why live if I'm not going to enjoy life? Besides, I'm Belgian. We use butter." She then stated, frowning, "I don't want to talk about this." When encouraged to tell me what might make it uncomfortable to talk about, she explained: "You're going to push me to follow my doctor's advice and I don't want to get into a fight with you." Claire's worry that

I'd push her might be partly a wish: Do you love me enough to fight for my survival? But it also represented a fear: Will you try to control me? Issues over autonomy were brought to life in the room with me.

Claire faced an important decision: Would she modify her diet to protect her health? Her worry that I would try to control her and her fear of our fighting echoed struggles for autonomy which had punctuated her childhood in rural Belgium. Claire had a devout, fearful mother who experienced her daughter's lively personality as evidence of the devil and therefore placed this daughter, at age 6, in a strict religious boarding school. Claire subsequently attended a series of such schools, for she excelled at getting herself expelled by defiantly breaking the rules. For example, she remembers telling one head priest that she did not believe in God and calling him to his face the French equivalent of "fatty." As we explored Claire's history, relational patterns of her childhood gradually become clear. For Claire, whose early ventures into self-expression were met punitively and by abandonment, the only way to experience autonomy was via defiant opposition. This opposition led to punishment but felt good. Now, once again, Claire was creating an oppositional relationship with an authority figure to experience autonomy.

For Claire the paradigmatic relationship contained one who dominated and one forced into shameful submission. She was determined never to be the one to submit. This relational pattern of Claire's was already known to her, for she had faced it in her analysis. Claire told me that her ease at taking a defiant stance had sometimes stood her in good stead. She attributed her success as a businesswoman in a man's field to that trait. But she recognized that this characterological pattern had also cost her dearly. Ruefully, she told me that it had led her to drop out of law school simply to spite her parents. And that it had destroyed her first marriage when, feeling controlled by her husband, she flouted her infidelity. "I worked through that pattern in my analysis," she told me. "I recognized what drove my need to defy others and eventually I became able to work for a boss, able to cooperate with my second husband." "But the fact is," she would add, "nobody can stop me from eating butter. I consider it an essential and I have the right to choose what I eat." As we explored this material, the developmental issues behind Claire's dilemma – whether to follow her doctor's advice – were becoming clearer. Claire's early struggle for autonomy and her early resolution of this struggle via defiance of authority, while worked through to some extent in her earlier analysis, had become alive again.

Claire's resolution of this dilemma began in a session when she told me about the joys of cooking with butter, the importance of the sensual pleasure of taste at a time of life when other pleasures had diminished, and her pride in her baking. She continued with a panegyric on the evils of diets and her hatred of vegetarians. "What do you hate about vegetarians?" I inquired. She told me at some length, concluding, "It's a religion for them. I hate that." As I listened, I associated to her troubled relationship with her mother, the mother who had tried to subdue her spirit by cramming religion down Claire's throat, by sending her off to a religious boarding school. So, I said to her something along the lines of: "I get it. A strict diet is like a strict religion. (Pause) If you follow your doctor's advice, if he and I end up coercing you into a restrictive diet, does that mean that your mother will finally have won? You will finally be forced to follow a religion?" I said this slowly and dramatically, using the kinds of intonations one adopts when reading to young children. I was not so much conveying information as telling a story. And it had quite an effect. Claire looked at me for a very long, astonished, pause – then erupted into peals upon peals of laughter. In her next sessions, she talked with tears about her coercive early environment and about how protesting harsh treatment had provided a way of keeping her soul alive. And we played together, making fun of the doctor/priest who was telling her what to eat and ordering her to kneel on rice as penance for her sins. Together we found hilarious ways of telling him to go to hell. What was the resolution? I knew Claire was beginning to find another mode of handling her needs for autonomy when she brought me a slice of her cake. "I made this with olive oil, not butter," she told me. "And it's actually pretty good." Her need to keep her soul alive by refusing to submit to the will of others was diminishing. Following her doctor's advice, no longer felt like "giving in." The cake, incidentally, was delicious.

Interpretation, long considered the major agent of change in psychoanalysis, plays a smaller role in treatment than previously thought. In this case with Claire, however, my interpretation had dramatic effects. I believe that it was not merely the content of this interpretation but also the emotional resonance evoked by the way I uttered it that accounted for its impact.

One of Claire's presenting problems was recent difficulty getting along with friends. She had friendships with a small circle of highly accomplished women who had been in her life for decades. Recently, she had been getting into fights with them. And now friends who had formerly loved spending summer weekends at her home on a lake in the country

were turning down invitations. As we explored this issue, I began to suspect that Claire's propensity for power struggles, the manifestation of her
crusade for autonomy, had always interfered with her friendships. The pattern she had revealed in our "battle of the butter," in which she would
experience humiliating subjugation if she allowed herself to be influenced
by me or her physician, was not new. With her internal template of what
Benjamin (1998) calls "doer/done to" relationships, she had probably
never cooperated easily. But now her pattern of interpersonal relating
had become more problematic, sufficiently so to endanger long-standing
friendships. What had happened?

As we reviewed her recent fights, Claire could see that she was being
"difficult." "I've always been difficult," she told me. "In fact, I've prided
myself on being a bit difficult. I'm a strong woman, not a pushover. But
I guess I might have gotten worse." Her suspicions were validated when
someone let slip that her friends were talking about her behind her back,
complaining to each other about how ornery she had become. She was
hurt when she learned of this. After discussing the problem with me, she
approached one friend and asked about it. Her friend told her the truth:
"I used to enjoy visiting you. I no longer do because you insist that I obey
your every command." Claire was stung by this, but also able to hear and
make use of it, bringing it to me to understand. "Do you think I've gotten
bossy?" she asked.

We then considered the many ways aging had eroded her sense of autonomy, her feelings of competence, her sense of self, and her identity. Claire
was no longer enjoying the feelings of accomplishment and success she
had gained in her business career. Crippling arthritis of her hands now
prevented her from working in her prizewinning garden. Although still an
attractive woman, she was no longer a magnet to men and felt the loss of
her sexual power keenly. Previously, she had filled the void left following her second husband's early death by having sexual relationships with
male friends. Now, she told me sadly, nobody was interested. She still had
sexual longings, but they remained unfulfilled. In a context of eroding
potency, perhaps she was unconsciously trying to restore it by becoming
controlling in her relationships and by being the "doer" rather than the
"done-to." We discussed this possibility.

Older adults sometimes make changes quickly. When Claire recognized
the nature of the trouble she was having in her relationships, she was determined to turn things around, and she jumped into action. After talking with
me about a recent skirmish with her daughter-in-law, for example, she

approached her, saying: "I've been thinking that I should stop telling you what to cook." It was not easy, and felt an affront to her pride, for Claire to admit that she might have played a part in the difficulty in their relationship. But she felt she needed to do that: "I'm too old to have time to fool around," she told me.

I doubt that Claire had a radical personality transformation. I suspect that she was still "difficult" in her relationships. But she was insightful about this problem and could use this insight when trouble brewed. Her pattern of needing control moderated enough that she began to enjoy her friendships again and was able once more to take pleasure in entertaining. Although she still lacked a sexual partner, she found herself relishing flirtatious encounters. Her depression lifted and she was enjoying life.

Then another issue from Claire's early years required our attention. I realized this only when exploring Claire's reactions to my summer vacation. With great shame, she confessed that she felt dependent on me, that she would not only miss me, but felt unsafe without me. We continued this exploration both before and after my vacation and a new side of Claire emerged. Her fear of conflict with me over the "butter" issue, she told me, was based on the dread that if she did not do what I told her to, I would kick her out of therapy. What emerged gradually was a terror of being abandoned. And memories returned of her anguish when she was first sent to boarding school. At the core of the belligerent hellion of her youth was a frightened child, believing it was her badness that had caused her abandonment. Her issues about autonomy were secondary to a profound lack of basic trust. Any false move and the unreliable other would discharge her, leaving her alone in her suffering. Her defiance was an example of "making passive active" (Fried, 1970), that is, of gaining a sense of control by precipitating what she feared would be done to her.

Understanding these feelings proved valuable in working on Claire's worries about death. Claire told me that since being told about her blocked carotid artery, she had become terrified at the prospect of dying. (Her defiant refusal to give up butter, I then realized, had been not only an attempt at autonomy but also a way to camouflage vulnerability – laughing in the face of death.) Together we explored these fears. It turned out that although an avowed atheist, Claire was worried that the religious teachings of her youth, beliefs she had long ago renounced, were true. Perhaps, as a sinner, she was doomed to an eternity in Hell. She would be alone, abandoned because of her misdeeds, subject to endless torment.

I have been influenced by Winnicott's (1974) teaching that the worst of what is feared is often the very thing that has already happened. And I have found that fantasized deaths sometimes contain images of past trauma. I agreed with Claire that neither of us knew what, if anything, happens after death and thus we had no way of knowing if the priests she had defied in childhood had been right all along. I acknowledged that I, too, feared death; also, that if the priests were correct, I, a Jew, would certainly end up in Hell. But I proposed a reason why Claire might have created that particular picture of death. The numerous separations during Claire's childhood had been punishments. She had been sent off to boarding school at a young age because she was "bad." Perhaps death, the ultimate separation, felt like a punishment. Claire was interested and acknowledged that the post-death feeling states she envisioned for herself were indeed like those she had experienced post-expulsion from home.

Making sense of these feelings did not, incidentally, erase Claire's fear of death, nor did I expect it to. One cannot analyze away fear of death. Putting emotions into words, sharing them with another, can, however, make them bearable (Glennon, 2016). Claire's fear of death did not disappear. But it receded further into the background and ceased dampening the pleasures of living.

After 4 years with me Claire was enjoying life. Although she got a lot out of seeing me, she told me, the round trip to and from Manhattan for our sessions was tiring and took time she needed for other activities. Although I knew there was more we could do, I also recognized how much we had done. She terminated her therapy with a twinkle in her eye.

References

Benjamin, J. (1998). *Shadow of the other: Intersubjectivity and gender in psychoanalysis.* Routledge.

Blatner, A. (1997). *Acting in: Practical application of psychodramatic methods* (3rd ed.). Free Association Press.

Blos, P. (1968). Character formation in adolescence. *Psychoanalytic Study of the Child, 23*, 245–263.

Erikson, E. H. (1984). Reflections on the last stage – And the first. *The Psychoanalytic Study of the Child, 39*, 155–165.

Erikson, E. H. (1998). *The life cycle completed,* Extended Version. W.W. Norton.

Freud, S. (1905). On psychotherapy. In J. Strachey (Ed. & Trans.), *The standard edition of the complete psychological works of Sigmund Freud* (Vol. 7, pp. 265–268). Hogarth Press.

Fried, E. (1970). *Active/passive: The crucial psychological dimension.* Grune & Stratton.

Gerson, M. J. (2018). Death of a parent: Openings at an ending. *Psychoanalytic Perspectives, 15*(3), 340–354.

Glennon, S.S. (2016). A courageous, creative, though cautionary tale: Commentary on Dr. Lauren Levine's paper, "A mutual survival of destructiveness and its creative potential for agency and desire." *Psychoanalytic Dialogues, 26*(1), 50–55.

Greenberg, T. M. (2016). *Psychodynamic perspective on aging and illness* (2nd ed.). Springer.

Kübler-Ross, E. (1969). *On death and dying.* Routledge.

Leveton, E. (1977). *Psychodrama for the timid clinician.* Springer Publishing Company.

Loewald, H. W. (1960). On the therapeutic action of psycho-analysis. *International Journal of Psycho-Analysis, 41,* 16–33.

Russell, P. L. (2006). The negotiation of affect. *Contemporary Psychoanalysis, 42*(4), 621–636.

Wagner, J. W. (2005). Psychoanalytic bias against the elderly patient: Hiding our fears under developmental millstones. *Contemporary Psychoanalysis, 41*(1), 77–92.

Winnicott, D. W. (1974). Fear of breakdown. *International Review of Psycho-Analysis, 1,* 103–107.

Chapter 3

Trauma and trauma redux

"I had a nightmare last night," Eliot told me. "I dreamed I was lying on a roof. And then I rolled off. I was falling. I was terrified and I told myself, 'Don't look down.' But I did look down and I kept saying to myself, 'There's supposed to be a safety net. There's supposed to be a safety net.' But there was no safety net. And then I woke up."

Eliot did lack a safety net. I was not providing him with one now, as he struggled with prostate cancer. Nor could his doctors guarantee his safety, although they were optimistic. But this was not the first time he had lacked a badly needed safety net. His childhood, adolescence, and early adulthood had been punctuated by traumatic episodes. And at these times, too, nobody had offered protection. Eliot's dream expressed a powerful mixture of feelings from both the past and the present. I will return to Eliot's story at the end of this chapter. I introduce his dream here to illustrate a frequently occurring phenomenon in older adults: the simultaneously experienced affects from both previous and current trauma.

Philip Roth (2007) described old age as not a battle but a massacre. In older age, it is not merely the fantasy of annihilation which is the problem. Rather, it is the imminence of actual annihilation. At any other stage of life something which will enfeeble you; kill off your spouse, siblings, and peers; assault you with physical discomfort if not outright agony; rob you of the activities which have given meaning to your life; and eventually assassinate you would be considered an unspeakable horror. In old age, simply because this is what happens to everybody, is it less than traumatic?

I will use the term "trauma" in discussing the ravages of older age. I am not arguing that the trauma faced by older adults is the same as that faced by people who suffered the Holocaust or whose villages were swept away by tsunamis. What I *am* saying is that many experiences of older adulthood can best be fathomed when identified as trauma. The disruptions to experiences of self, the terror of immediate extinction, the collapse of symbolization, the reckoning with contingency, and the fear of disintegration of the body – these are the experiences of older adults which can best be understood through the lens of trauma. In addition, the therapeutic action of the psychodynamic treatment of older adults can best be understood when concepts developed in treating trauma are added to those more traditional in psychodynamic work. And, finally, the transference–countertransference configurations that arise in this work may resemble those described in the treatment of trauma survivors.

What is trauma? And is it legitimate to apply the concept of trauma to the ordinary experiences of older age? Definitions of trauma often include pre-cipitating events, such as threatened death, risk to physical safety, or wit-nessing the deaths of others (e.g., American Psychiatric Association, 2013). They may include the effects on the individual caused by these events, such as entering a state of extreme helplessness, of the fissure of experi-ence, and of dissociation (e.g., Howell & Itzkowitz, 2016). And definitions may require that the events involved be at the extremes of experience, far beyond what is ordinarily expectable in life (e.g., Boulanger, 2007).

The hardships older adults face frequently encompass most, if not all, of these aspects of trauma. To older adults, the threat of death and disability is a constant. In addition, many elders suffer states of helplessness and anguish which lead to either emotional flooding and agitation or a dead-ened, dissociative state. And while it is true that the vicissitudes of older age are not extreme, that they happen to all of us if we reach old age and are therefore expectable, it is not necessarily true that we expect them. Such is the power of what Becker (1973) calls the "denial of death" that we know, but at the same time may not know, that we will die. Intellectu-ally, death may be expectable; emotionally, it may not. Stolorow (2007) discusses the "absolutisms" in daily life, which provide "a kind of naïve realism and optimism that allow one to function in the world, experienced as stable and predictable" (p. 16). Trauma, he tells us, deconstructs these absolutisms, bringing the recognition that reality is random and unpredict-able. Older age does the same and, in that way, may traumatize.

In applying trauma theory to the treatment of older adults, I start with the writings of Boulanger (2007). She makes a distinction between the effects of early vs. adult-onset trauma, believing, as I do, that these two are not mutually exclusive. When children are traumatized, she states, the result is the sequestration of these experiences into split off, dissociated self-states. Adult-onset trauma, on the other hand, results in damage to what she calls the "core self." The sense of self then collapses, is radically altered. Older patients, I have found, often exhibit the effects of both late-onset and early trauma. The traumatizing events they undergo in their current lives often have a sizable impact on the core self. At the same time, present-day trauma often triggers trauma from previous years, sparking to life long-sequestered emotional states. Previously dissociated experiences are relived as if happening now. Thus, people in their later years may suffer doubly. The twofold origin of their distress not only challenges the clinician but also provides opportunity. For in facing the torments of the past and present simultaneously, in finding words for and coming to understand and to metabolize the sensations, feelings, and memories which are evoked by the experiences of older age, in many cases individuals arrive at more integrated and nuanced self-narratives, at more robust and positive senses of self, and at more affectively whole states of being than they experienced earlier in their lives. The greater insight into self and self-in-relationship achieved in this way may also allow a depth of working through of relational conflicts previously unattainable. Even people who benefitted greatly from previous therapy may be astonished by their own late-life flowering, as they find themselves able to make strides in dealing with issues they have struggled with for decades. In addition, since having an integrated self and self-narrative helps greatly in finding meaning and therefore also in facing death, this work brings many rewards. It is not unusual for an older patient – even ones beset by considerable current hardship – to say, "You know, I'm the best I've ever been."

In this chapter, I will start by looking at the way the traumatizing experiences of older age affect the core self. I will then move to the way these experiences can also evoke trauma from earlier times. I will continue to a brief discussion of the effectiveness of psychodynamic psychotherapy in the simultaneous treatment of past and current trauma. I will conclude by returning to my work with Eliot, illustrating the way the treatment of both types of trauma can contribute not only to a reduction in suffering but also to new growth, to psychological advancement.

Late-onset trauma in older adults

The aspects of the core self which Boulanger describes as severely disrupted in late-onset trauma are agency, physical cohesion, continuity, and affectivity. All these disruptions to the core self can be found in older adults.

The core self: agency

The sense of agency, of being in control of one's body, of making choices, and of being the composer of the symphony of one's life – this is usually considered an important feature of mental health. The psychotherapy patient who lacks the experience of self-as-agent is what Schafer (1983) describes as "the imprisoned analysand" and is missing an important ingredient in a good life. Whereas individuals subjected to catastrophic events may lose their sense of agency in one episode of horror, agency in older age is eroded by a thousand small cuts. Over time, increasingly: one's body does not obey; one's mind fails to retrieve or retain; and one's choices are ever more limited. Control of one's body, mind, and life must be ceded to the realities of one's biology.

Sid, an 83-year-old, tells me: "My eye doctor took away my right to drive. Since my prostate operation, I can't control my pee. Even with my hearing aids, I can't participate in a conversation in a restaurant. When I meet old friends on the street, I can't recall their names. And I'm spending down my money instead of earning it. I'm a disaster." Sid's experience as an agentic self has been severely compromised by the "normal" events of aging.

The core self: cohesion of the body

Cohesion of the body is one of the background assumptions that contribute to a sense of groundedness in the self and in the life. But bodies are fragile and disruptions to the body can have a strong impact on the sense of self. In Conway's words (2007), "Damage to the body constitutes damage to the self" (p. 42). In a catastrophic event, the experience of cohesion of the body can be pierced in an instant. In contrast, as one ages, it often diminishes in a long slow arc. In medical settings, major organs of the body are scrutinized, scanned, biopsied, and possibly removed. In the gym, ligaments are torn, backs go into spasm, and muscles refuse to cooperate. In the home, jars refuse to open, genitals function only with medical intervention, mirrors reveal wrinkles, and every area rug becomes a potential bonebreaker. There are daily reminders of the dissolution of the body. In addition, the ultimate destroyer of body, death, can no longer be denied. The numerous assaults to the cohesion of the body may erode the experience of a cohesive self.

Sarah, a 77-year-old widow, tells me, "Yesterday I had trouble getting down the subway stairs because my left leg kept buckling. I got terrified that I'm going to need a knee replacement. Then at home I saw that more of my hair has been falling out. I tried to calm myself with a glass of wine, but my hands were too weak to open the bottle. I used to be able to count on my body. What's happened?" For Sarah, the self-experience that is rooted in having an intact, working body has been badly shaken.

The core self: going on being

A third aspect of the core self is what Winnicott (1975) called "going on being," the sense of being the same self through the past, present, and future, of self-continuity. But, in Slochower's (2019) words, he failed to discuss "our adult vulnerability to the *real* ending of our going on being" (p. 550). The sense of going on being can be greatly altered in later life. Typically, adults inhabit what Bach (2008) terms "analog states," in which they experience "a continuity in their life because at any given moment they know where they have come from and can imagine where they are going" (p. 785). He contrasts this with trauma-induced "digital states," in which "the experience of life is a succession of instantaneous digital moments, without connection to or even memory of where they have come from and where they might be going." In these latter states people feel "vulnerable and uprooted as if they were constantly balancing on one foot." For many older adults, the self may be experienced as timeless – but then something comes to disrupt, propelling them into Bach's digital states. The disrupting event may be as trivial, but jarring, as a glance in the mirror, leading to: "I'm the same me I've always been. So, who is that old lady in the mirror? This can't be me." In other cases, larger life events disrupt the sense of continuity with the past, demolishing old identities. Retirement can destroy a robust work-self. The loss of a spouse can disorder self-experience because "suddenly the self-with-other identity has been supplanted by a self that is without" (Aragno, 2007, p. 35). Meanwhile, the sense of continuity with the future is sharply curtailed by the acute awareness that death may, at any moment and without warning, end it all. Past and future are disconnected, and the sense of "going on being" may deteriorate.

Howard, bedridden, comments: "I can no longer connect with the me who went to work every day, ran marathons and reveled in hot sex. Who is this old man with one foot in the grave who can barely make it to the bathroom? This isn't me." Howard's experience of "going on being" has been deeply disturbed by his current life situation. His identities as a worker, athlete, and lover have been stripped away, weakening his connection with his past self, while his sense of approaching death deprives him of contact with an envisioned future self.

The core self: affectivity

In the Darwinian struggle for survival mammals are hardwired to fight to stay alive. Their biology privileges reactivity to stimuli which evoke threats to survival, and they will prepare to fight or to flee when beset by such stimuli. The roar of a lion will send deer running. But what about humans? We have the same reactions to that which could kill us. We have the same physiological responses (e.g., activation of the sympathetic nervous system and secretion of cortisol) as other mammals when we recognize danger. But in contrast to other animals, we also know that we will die. We learn this early – just how early is a surprising result of research on young children. Solomon et al. (2015) describe studies identifying worries about death in children as young as three and five. They also report on research in which, contrary to their mothers' predictions, 8–12-year-olds stated that they were more afraid of death than of snakes or of bad report cards. The human organism faces the reality/danger of death in the absence of the lion's roar. How humans manage their knowledge of their mortality has been the subject of much thought by philosophers, theologians, anthropologists, psychologists, and psychoanalysts, and there are many aspects to this question. (These will be discussed more in Chapter 6.) Most relevant here is the way the knowledge of impending death may affect the affectively grounded sense of self of the older adult. For in older age, the most common mode of managing death anxiety, denial, crumbles. And the resulting terror can overwhelm.

In some cases, it leads to a chronic state of anxiety and agitation. In many others, it leads to numbness and an accompanying loss of subjective aliveness. Deadness "can be the last alternative to profound fear" Chefetz (2015, p. 178). Other affects such as intense grief, excruciating regret, envy, or rage may contribute to numbing. One's affective being, overloaded by the unbearable, may shut down. But to live fully, one must bear one's unbearable affects. In a numb, deadened state, the core self, which requires the experience of aliveness and an ongoing connection with feeling, may collapse.

Harriet tells me: "I'm waiting for the results of my biopsy and I still can't believe my husband's diagnosis. I should feel afraid or angry or sad. Instead I feel absolutely nothing. I guess I'm dead inside." Harriet has lost contact with an affective self.

Given these assaults on the core selves of the aged – on their agency, bodily cohesion, continuity, and affectivity – even people who have had relatively stable senses of self when younger may lose that in older age. This kind of disruption to the self is well described by Alpert (2012), an analyst who endured a 12-year marathon of watching her husband felled and eventually killed by a degenerative neurological disease. Although she is reporting on the psychic effects of chronic illness, her words are readily applicable to the experiences of the aged as they react to drastic changes in their bodies. Alpert identifies a process she names, "loss of humanness." In her words "there is talk of body parts as if they are separate from themselves. It is as if, in that moment, they are looking at some part of themselves as belonging in the after while they are in the before. The lived past and the ongoing present are different. They feel as if they have lost part of themselves or, perhaps, their whole selves" (p. 124).

One of the goals of therapy for older adults is to help restore the self in the face of decimating assault. This task, however, is complicated by a second hazard: For many, the traumatic experiences of old age may call to life earlier traumatic experiences. When that happens, therapy requires working with the trauma of the past and present simultaneously.

Trauma redux

"One feels inclined to doubt sometimes whether the dragons of primaeval days are really extinct," wrote Freud (1937, p. 385). A more contemporary version of that understanding was penned by Stolorow (2015): "Trauma recovery is an oxymoron" (p. 134). Encoded in neural networks, early experiences of trauma never disappear. Childhood traumatic experiences that are too overwhelming to be assimilated are dissociated, becoming self-states which remain unknown, unlinked to other experience (Howell & Itzkowitz, 2016). These early experiences are not remembered; they are so split off that they cannot be accessed via association. How, then, can we come to know them? One method used by psychoanalysts is recognizing them through their expression in enactments. In these, patient and therapist, unawares, co-participate in complex behaviors which manifest dissociated aspects of both parties (Bromberg, 2011). Analyzing these enactments leads to insight into the patient's long-buried early traumatic experience. There is, in addition, a second gateway to these earlier traumatic experiences: When current sensation replicates early sensation, memories, sensations, and affects from earlier phases of life may come flooding back. A horrific example is reported by Brenner (2020): Physical restraint required to keep his father safe while in a ventilator caused him to relive the long-dissociated trauma of being buried alive during the Holocaust. Oncologists recognize that having a life-threatening diagnosis may rouse past demons – bringing back, for example, the memories and feelings of an early rape (Sekeres, 2019). Old age is, in one sense, a life-threatening diagnosis and can rouse the demons.

Many older adults have suffered some degree of early relational trauma and carry with them corresponding sequelae, dissociated self-states. Given enough strength and sufficiently benign circumstances, they may have built reasonably good lives for themselves, lives in which their pockets of pain seldom caused distress. And then come the ravages of older age, when the sensations accompanying new trauma can trigger old trauma. Then even individuals who have successfully navigated long lives with sealed off earlier trauma may find themselves persecuted by the ghosts of these early happenings, as described in Chapter 2. Physical illness, unrelenting pain, loss of attachment figures, isolation, experiences rendering one helpless, and terror of death – these can trigger the affects and memories of early ordeals. These cause self-states to "break out of their dissociated captivity" (Bromberg, 2011, p. 5), and early experiences are relived as if happening now.

Memory researchers are now studying that phenomenon, reporting that current stimuli can bring up intrusive affects from past trauma in a process they call "reexperiencing" (Ehlers, 2015). In reexperiencing, stimuli accompanying a current situation which match the stimuli of a traumatizing experience of the past can evoke an unbidden memory with considerable emotional impact (Berntsen, 2015). When this happens, the affects or physiological reactions from the past trauma can be reexperienced without the awareness that they stem from a traumatic memory. In Siegel's (2020) words, "Implicit memory does not have a sense of 'something being remembered'" (p. 142). Thus, the emotional experience of the present may not be recognized as a visitor from the past but instead attributed to the events of the present. The revived trauma is experienced as if it is currently happening.

Let me insert a note of caution here. It is crucial in treating those suffering the simultaneous effects of both current and revived trauma that one does not simply ascribe current pain to events of the past. Unfortunately, a traditionally psychodynamic approach can be, indeed has been, misused by this type of intervention, one harmful to older patients. What happens in old age is all too real and to interpret the distress arising from these incidents as solely a product of the past can be both invalidating and a denial of reality. At the same time, locating the source of distress as only in the present can also be problematic. For the meaning one gives a painful event greatly influences how it is experienced and because emotions and self-experiences of past trauma can infiltrate the present. The influence of past and present co-exist in dialectical tension and both must be taken into account.

Here are some examples of sensations activating old trauma. Urinary incontinence, with its dreaded sensation of warm, wet urine saturating undergarments, for example, may arouse shameful feelings from childhood "accidents" that were harshly punished or ridiculed. Needing a helping hand after falling may bring back emotions stemming from times when pleas for help were met with angry slaps and derisive comments. The pain from arthritis or surgery may recall the agony of childhood beatings. The death of a spouse may revive a traumatic early abandonment. In addition, the insults of ageism can revive early experiences of being treated with contempt. Intense shame and self-loathing, the experience of badness, of unlovability, and of deserving to suffer, feeling isolated as if suspended alone in outer space, helplessness in the face of powerful persecuting others, and terror – these are the kinds of dissociated emotions from the distant past which can be awakened by current hardship and can color current affective states. Thus, the clinician facing the suffering older adult often must find a way to treat the simultaneous presence of both past and current trauma. How do we do that?

How psychotherapy can help

How can psychotherapy help an individual whose core self has been severely disrupted by the traumatizing experiences of older age and who is suffering revived early trauma? We cannot stop the assaults on the core self which are precipitated by the rigors of aging. That is, we cannot prevent "hits" to agency, bodily cohesion, the sense of going on being, and affectivity. And we cannot ward off revived early trauma. As it happens, many components of psychodynamic psychotherapy are helpful in the restoration of the cohesion of the core self and in the reduction of suffering occasioned by the combined trauma of past and present.

Bolstering the core self

Agency

Older adults may have reduced ability to experience agency via having an impact in the world or via control of the body. But they can enhance their sense of agency by their ability to transform their inner landscapes. Their work in therapy can bring a sense of mastery and delight as they make connections and gain new understandings of themselves and others. It can lead them to "try out" new behaviors in relationships. Ways of relating to others previously unimaginable may become available: asking for help directly, expressing gratitude and affection, and self-assertion. Older adults then experience themselves as still capable of growth and as agents of their own change. The therapy process can also arouse their curiosity leading to interest in themselves and their own experience of aging. They can see themselves as explorers discovering new truths. As Buechler (2019) puts it, "Aging can occasion exciting adventures as we discover our own hidden depth" (p. 59). The undertaking of this journey can help restore the agentic self.

Ruth exclaims: "Sunday I found myself telling my grandson that I love him. And I saw his face light up. You may not get what a big deal that is. I always hated being 'sentimental.' Knowing about my family, you understand why. But this time I was able to say it, to enjoy saying it, and to marvel at what it meant to him. Isn't it amazing that at this age I can still change!" Ruth is experiencing her agency.

Cohesion of the body

Talk therapy cannot alter the trajectory of bodily decline in older patients and, therefore, the older adults may be deprived of the grounding of self-experience which stems from having a robust body. Nevertheless, much can be done to restore the sense of a bodily self. The process of talking about physical changes, mourning the loss of the younger body, and appreciating and caring for the existing body – these all foster the integration of the body-of-the-present into the sense of self. Bringing into awareness and countering social stereotypes which include the equation "old = ugly" aids in this process of reclaiming a sense of the body's goodness. Helping patients focus less on appearance and instead on the body as sensed and felt fosters the capacity for the experience of an embodied self (Sands, 2020). Recognizing and working with the unconscious meaning of body parts, bodily functions, and physical impairments can also be helpful. If, for example, a patient's firm, toned body was experienced as a representation of efficacy, of self-discipline, or of overcoming vulnerability, the loss of muscle tone may be experienced as a drastic diminishment of the self. Making sense of these meanings can help the impact of bodily change become less injurious to the self.

Peter tells me: "I just realized why I'm so upset about my knee being out of whack, why I can't tolerate hobbling with a cane. Of course, I can't stand people looking at me and feeling sorry for me. But, also, being able to run away saved me from my father's drunken attacks. For me, being able to move fast has always protected me from mistreatment and has represented safety. Once I realized that, I had to laugh. As an adult, there are lots of other things I can do. I can talk with a sharp tongue, complain to the Better Business bureau, or even call the police. I don't need to run to be safe."

Affectivity

As Berzoff (2019) puts it, "There is something about sharing the pain in a therapeutic encounter, however intense it might be, which helps it become bearable" (p. 125). There is probably a neurological role in this effect, since neurologist note that we function as external neural circuits for one another (Cozolino, 2008). When we join our patients in their dark states and feel with them, they can weather their agonizing feelings. This is the aspect of witnessing which Eshel (2016) calls "withnessing." Our emotionally engaged presence alters the nature of the patient's experience and in this way a patient's state of emotional deadness can be replaced by aliveness – aliveness-with-pain, it is true, but freedom from deadness. In the process the patient's experience as an emotional being revives and the capacity to experience intense feeling expands.

In addition, our work may alter patients' relationships with their own affectivity. For many, the experience of intense emotion is accompanied by unformulated negative self-evaluations. Thus, the sense of self is eroded not only by the shutting down of unbearable emotion but also by self-judgment of this emotion. We are all affected by what Buechler (2019) calls, "a culturally scripted idealization of stoicism" (p. 45). Our society tells us we should triumph over negative feelings. A striking example, memorable to those of a certain age, is the outpouring of praise Jackie Kennedy received for managing not to cry during the tragedy of her husband's funeral. In addition, judgment of affect may stem from family prohibitions. The narcissistic mother described by Alice Miller (1981) may be so wounded by her child's unhappiness that she sends the message, "Your sad feelings are an attack on me." Psychotherapy fosters the development of what Jurist (2018) calls "mentalized affectivity," insight into one's emotional experience. The perspective gained can transform one's relationship to one's emotions.

Sue questions what is wrong with her that she still weeps over her husband's death eight months ago. I tell her that weeping is not a weakness. Together we explore the experiences which have led her to believe that she should be "over it," that her sadness is pathological. Gradually, she is able to continue weeping with less self-judgment.

Going on being

Much of what we do is help patients tell, and enrich the telling of, their stories. We hear the stories of their lives and work with them to fill in the blanks – the blanks left by that which is not consciously available, by what was never formulated (Stern, 1997), by what they were not allowed to know, and by what was split off. As I will discuss further in Chapter 5, recognizing patterns, making meaning, identifying feelings and putting them into words, and gaining an autobiographical perspective on the course of a long life – all these activities knit together the past and present and strengthen the sense of self-continuity.

Raymond says, "Gosh, I had forgotten all this stuff I'm telling you about how I managed to work my way through graduate school. I guess I'm using what I learned then to work my way through cancer. I may be falling apart physically, but I haven't changed that much!"

Recognizing past trauma as past

As tormenting as reliving early trauma can be, this reliving provides opportunity by making long-sequestered, dissociated experiences available for examination. Sometimes, detailed memories emerge. Sometimes, it is merely the old feelings that surface. As they find words for and metabolize the sensations and feelings evoked by the experiences of older age and as they integrate them into autobiographical memory, patients recognize the way the experiences of the present are haunted by past trauma. This can weaken the grip of past trauma on the sense of self, reducing shame, and the sense of isolation.

Susan, age 84, had forgotten to sign a financial form, precipitating a cash flow problem for the next month. Flooded with fear, she could barely verbalize what the problem was. I knew that Susan had financial concerns and that she worried whether her savings were sufficient to see her through the rest of her life. But I also guessed that there were simple solutions to her current problem, that she could simply move money between accounts. I also knew that in her career she had managed a large agency budget. What could account for her current terrorized state? Since she grew up in a family often "on welfare," I ask her if the worries about money then might be affecting her now. She was intrigued, became somewhat calmer, and told me that she wanted to think about that. She started her next session, telling me:

> You were right. I've always remembered how poor we were – how we used cardboard to fix holes in our shoes. But I never remembered the feelings. Last week I was remembering those feelings. No, actually I was feeling the feelings. I felt terrified and a memory came back. I remembered that when my kid sister was born, I overheard my mother say to a neighbor, "We have no money, so I'm not sure we'll be able to keep her." After that, every time we were short of money, I got frightened that I'd be sent away. I walked around terrified a lot of the time. I had forgotten those feelings.

Susan then added,

> Of course, as an adult I've been short of money at times, but then
> I could always take on a second job to see me through. I did that more
> than once. This time, I realized that there was no getting a second job.
> If I ran out of money, I was sunk. That's why I was so frightened.

Susan's panic is an example of reexperiencing. Emotions of the past,
revived by current stimuli, were relived in the present. The feelings aroused
were not recognized as stemming from a memory but were instead attributed to events of the present. The dangers she had faced as a child were felt
as if they were present now. And the defenses she had developed to counter those overwhelming feelings – empowering herself by moving into
action and finding a second job – were no longer available to her. Susan's
recall of the childhood experience that had terrified her and her connecting
her current affective state with this memory was helpful, relieving.

Eliot: treating trauma and trauma redux in combination

I return now to Eliot, who dreamed of rolling off a roof. Our work illustrates the way past and present trauma can be woven together by life's
circumstances – and the value of recognizing and treating both.

Eliot, a gay musician in his 70s, started therapy with me for depression
when in his early 60s. We worked then on issues of submission to and
caretaking of others. We worked on his chronic shame and the way he hid
his inner life from others to stay safe, despite yearnings for greater closeness. Then, because of a geographical move initiated by his ill partner,
Eliot left earlier than either of us felt ideal. He had come a long way, but
there were still issues which needed work. Eliot had been sexually absti-
nent for decades. He and his partner were in a nonsexual relationship,
preceding which he had been celibate for many years. He felt starved for
a more intimate relationship, and he yearned to do more with his music.

After his partner died, Eliot returned and we resumed twice weekly therapy.
Initially we were immersed in his grief: grief over his recent loss and grief
revived over the loss of the gay community, the community decimated by
HIV, which had sustained him during early adulthood. He began to feel better.
He would say, "I'm not happy, but I'm content." Then he was diagnosed with

prostate cancer and entered a profound, deadened depression with suicidal ideation – a depression unrelieved by antidepressant medication.

Still bereft by the loss of his partner, a man who had succumbed to the ravages of cancer, Eliot knew all too well what the worst-case scenario might be. Although his doctor, citing the results of scans and tests, was optimistic, he expected the worst. Here are the kinds of things he said at those times: "My life is, and always will be, run by cancer. It will never go away." "Who knows how bad the damage to my body will be, what they'll do surgically, what the meds will do to me." "I know this is nuts, but I can't make any plans, since I don't believe I have a future." "The things I used to look forward to and which have always given me pleasure no longer do." These feelings reveal the extent to which the prostate cancer diagnosis and treatment constituted a traumatic assault on his core self. For the very aspects of the core self which Boulanger (2007) states are disrupted by late-life trauma – the senses of agency, of bodily cohesion, of self-continuity, and of affectivity – were indeed disrupted.

The cancer diagnosis and treatment represented real, current trauma. But in addition to these reactions, Eliot now suffered intense feelings which stemmed from earlier trauma, much of which impinged on genitals, sexuality and his sense of masculinity. From his youngest years, he had been bullied by a brother who would beat him up, pin him down, and render him powerless. Nobody ever came to help. At age 7, he had been hospitalized for genital surgery. With a family too repressed about sexual matters to answer his questions, he believed that he was permanently damaged. (This experience, incidentally, was so dissociated that it only emerged as a "recovered memory" decades later, at which time Eliot was able to get confirmation of its validity from family members.) Then at age 12, he was violently raped by a teenaged boy. Sexually excited, he was also helpless and terrified, believing that he would die. He left the experience feeling dirty and degraded. His shame was such that he never revealed this to a soul, including two former therapists, until he was finally able to tell me. Meanwhile, he struggled, as teen boys of his generation did, to understand his non-hetero-normative sexual responses in a homophobic world. Subsequently, entering gay life in NYC, he was assaulted by an older man who got him drunk and forcibly raped him. Then, during the AIDS crisis, he lost many of his friends and lovers at a time when sex could mean death. In addition, I am saddened to say, when he sought help, he went through a 6- or 7-year psychoanalysis aimed at changing his sexual orientation – an analysis which further reinforced his self-experience of defectiveness.

The diagnosis of prostate cancer and subsequent medical procedures entailed genitals being handled by medical personnel, confusing and painful physical sensations, the fear that the source of sexual excitement was also lethal, feeling at the mercy of cancer, and the sense that death was imminent. These experiences were traumatizing in themselves. But in the same way that a car backfiring can catapult a traumatized veteran back into a war zone, they also revived the affects from earlier trauma. Eliot felt intense shame, a self-experience as unattractive and intellectually inferior, of having nothing to offer, of being insufficiently masculine, sexually unappealing and defective. He also felt terrorized and helpless. These feelings sprang from the cancer and also from earlier trauma.

I told Eliot that in addition to the misery caused by the current trauma of prostate cancer, he might also be reexperiencing the feelings from past trauma. He was intrigued and became curious about what he was feeling. Although he continued to suffer, he felt at least a modicum of relief. This emotional shift is a good example of how one emotion can modulate another (Buechler, 2008). Eliot's distress was at least slightly moderated by his accompanying curiosity. Our work then took place on two levels. We continued to recognize the impact of the roller coaster of cancer treatment and screenings. And we worked at putting into words and understanding the feelings from earlier trauma. This was not easy for either of us, for we were immersed in feeling states that frequently felt unbearable. Then all this work would shift into the background as we dealt with new medical results, new scares, and the frustrations of dealing with a dysfunctional medical system. We would talk about death, his fears of it, my acknowledgment that I struggle with it, too. I would worry about losing him and he would feel he needed to take care of me, as he had taken care of his mother, by not worrying me. Thus, the work continued.

Depression may be the product of dissociated shame (Bose, 2016). Eliot's traumatic experiences had resulted in considerable shame, especially over sexuality. "Left unrepaired, the disintegrating experience of shame will become a chronic state of self," states DeYoung (2015, p. 140). Eliot's self-disgust, his need to hide, and his long-term sexual abstinence were manifestations of this shame. The sensations surrounding prostate cancer and its treatment brought into awareness long-dissociated, powerful experiences of shame which could now be put into words and made explicable.

The fruits of this labor have been a source of real joy. Eliot is no longer depressed, although, in the context of his medical situation we cannot prevent his suffering. He does have his bad days. But, as a result of our intersubjective processing of raw affect from both past and present, he can bear this distress without numbing himself. Although he has deep regrets and mourns what could have been, he can also appreciate the goodness of his previous life and has regained contact with the parts of himself that he likes. This has allowed him the further working through of long-standing relational issues. He has moved from relationships in which he either served as caretaker to or was dominated by others to ones more mutual. He speaks up more freely and is sometimes surprised at his own willingness to reveal feelings and experiences which he formerly hid. His relationships, he tells me, are the best they've ever been. In fact, he's the best he's ever been.

Eliot has become more creative and productive in his life as a musician. With newfound leadership ability, he has taken on key roles in an organization which contributes to its surrounding community. In addition, he recently had a sexual encounter – an intensely gratifying one – the first in nearly 40 years. In his next session, he told me, "I realized I would give up everything just for the smell of him." And then, with gut-wrenching sobs, he expressed his intense grief over the long sexless decades of his life and his rage at the psychoanalyst who had intensified his internalized homophobia. Eliot emerged from this experience with a newly acquired hope of having the relationship he yearns for. Meanwhile, however, we live through ups and downs as he undergoes medical scrutiny; our awareness of mortality is a constant presence. Our work continues, painful at times, yet also enlivening and enriching.

References

Alpert, J. L. (2012). Loss of humanness: The ultimate trauma. *The American Journal of Psychoanalysis, 72*(2), 118–138.

American Psychiatric Association. (2013). *Diagnostic and statistical manual of mental disorders* (5th ed.). American Psychiatric Association.

Aragno, A. (2007). Transforming mourning: A new psychoanalytic perspective. In B. Willock, L. C. Bohm, & R. C. Curtis (Eds.), *On deaths and endings: Psychoanalysts' reflections on finality, transformations and new beginnings* (pp. 21–41). Routledge.

Bach, S. (2008). On digital consciousness and psychic death. *Psychoanalytic Dialogues, 18*(6), 784–794.

Becker, E. (1973). *The denial of death*. Free Press.

Berntsen, D. (2015). From everyday life to trauma: Research on everyday involuntary memories advances our understanding of intrusive memories of trauma. In L. A. Watson & D. Berntsen (Eds.), *Clinical perspectives on autobiographical memory* (pp. 172–196). Cambridge University Press.

Berzoff, J. (2019). Being still: Sitting with suffering in long-term relational practice. In S. A. Lord (Ed.), *Reflections on long-term relational psychotherapy and psychoanalysis: Relational analysis interminable* (pp. 119–131). Routledge.

Bose, J. (2016). Dissociative process and the depressed patient. *Contemporary Psychoanalysis, 52*(1), 51–75.

Boulanger, G. (2007). *Wounded by reality: Understanding and treating adult onset trauma*. Routledge.

Brenner, I. (2020). The last witnesses: Learning about life and death from aging survivors. *International Journal of Psychoanalysis, 101*(2), 340–354.

Bromberg, P. M. (2011). *The shadow of the tsunami and the growth of the relational mind*. Routledge.

Buechler, S. (2008). *Making a difference in patients' lives: Emotional experience in the therapeutic setting*. Routledge.

Buechler, S. (2019). *Psychoanalytic approaches to problems in living: Addressing life's challenges in clinical practice*. Routledge.

Chefetz, R. A. (2015). *Intensive psychotherapy for persistent dissociative processes: The fear of feeling real*. W.W. Norton.

Conway, K. (2007). *Illness and the limits of expression*. University of Michigan Press.

Cozolino, L. (2008). *The healthy aging brain: Sustaining attachment, attaining wisdom*. W.W. Norton.

DeYoung, P. A. (2015). *Understanding and treating chronic shame: A relational/neurological approach*. Routledge.

Ehlers, A. (2015). Intrusive reexperiencing in posttraumatic stress disorder: Memory process and their implications for therapy. In L. A. Watson & D. Berntsen (Eds.), *Clinical perspectives on autobiographical memory* (pp. 109–132). Cambridge University Press.

Eshel, O. (2016). The "voice" of breakdown" On facing the unbearable traumatic experience in psychoanalytic work. *Contemporary Psychoanalysis, 52*(1), 76–110.

Freud, S. (1937). Analysis terminable and interminable. *International Journal of Psychoanalysis, 18*, 373–405.

Howell, E. F., & Itzkowitz, S. (2016). The everywhereness of trauma and the dissociative structuring of the mind. In E. F. Howell & S. Itzkowitz (Eds.), *The dissociative mind in psychoanalysis: Understanding and working with trauma* (pp. 33–43). Routledge.

Jurist, E. (2018). *Minding emotions: Cultivating mentalization in psychotherapy*. Guilford Press.

Miller, A. (1981). *Prisoners of childhood*. Basic Books.

Roth, P. (2007). *Everyman*. Knopf Doubleday.

Sands, S. H. (2020). Body experience in the analysis of the older woman. *Psychoanalytic Inquiry, 40*(3), 173–188.

Schafer, R. (1983). *The analytic attitude*. Basic Books.

Sekeres, M. A. (2019, January 1). What lies beneath the surface. *New York Times*, p. D4.

Siegel, D. J. (2020). *The developing mind: How relationships and the brain interact to shape who we are*. Guilford Press.

Slochower, J. (2019). Getting better all the time? *Psychoanalytic Dialogues, 29*(5), 548–559.

Solomon, S., Greenberg, J., & Pyszczynski, T. (2015). *The worm at the core: On the role of death in life*. Penguin Books.

Stern, D. B. (1997). *Unformulated experience: From dissociation to imagination in psychoanalysis*. Analytic Press.

Stolorow, R. D. (2007). *Trauma and human existence: Autobiographical, psychoanalytic and philosophical reflections*. Routledge.

Stolorow, R. D. (2015). A phenomenological-contextual, existential and ethical perspective on emotional trauma. *Psychoanalytic Review, 102*(1), 123–138.

Winnicott, D. W. (1975). *Through pediatrics to psychoanalysis*. Basic Books.

Chapter 4

Dramatis personae, past and present

A painful but educative incident

Her voice cracked with fury and her face reddened with rage. "You're trying to kill me," she screamed. Frieda turned on me and continued in that vein and at that volume for several minutes. I was a disgrace, she told me. How dare I call myself a psychologist, when I clearly didn't care about the people I work with. She had been fooled by me. She had thought that I was a kind person and that she was special to me. Now she knew the truth. Now she knew that I was a selfish bitch. Now she knew that I was there for her money. She became silent and glared.

I sat stunned, trying to quiet my racing pulse. I knew enough to remain still until I could address this calmly. And, silently, I thought about what had just transpired. What had I done to elicit this attack? I had come to work that day with a cold – with a raspy voice, a cough, and an adjacent box of tissues. In her eyes, this was murderous, exploitive behavior. My mind flashed to a psychiatric inpatient I had once worked with who, in a psychotic break, thought I was trying to poison him. But I knew that she was not psychotic. So, what was happening here?

I knew that Frieda had what her friends and family described as "a temper problem," a descriptive term she attributed to their judgmental response when a woman expressed herself honestly. I knew that she had a way of organizing experience into extremes of good and bad, where all was black or white, never gray. I knew that she was shouting at me in the voice that had been used on her in her abusive childhood home. And I knew, I was experiencing the relational pattern that I had previously recognized in her relationships with others: her handling feelings of vulnerability by engaging in brutal combat. I knew that it was important for us to understand this.

I, therefore, did what my psychoanalytic training had taught me to do and inquired more about her experience. She told me and I listened. We discussed my behavior and its effect on her. I did not become defensive; I merely tried to explore fully what this had meant to her. But here's the thing. As I listened, I was sure I had done nothing wrong. Yes, I had come to work with a cold. But I always worked through colds, as did most of my colleagues. Unless I had a fever, I never stayed home. Internally, although I said nothing about this, I assumed she was experiencing me as her abusive parent. Although contemporary psychoanalytic theory had taught me that there is no blank screen, that the therapist is a participant in the patient's transference, I believed I was innocent: Her parent was the guilty party. And Frieda, no fool, recognized my internal stance. I am grateful to her for sticking with this process and eventually remarking on my lack of remorse. In this way, she brought something important to my awareness. It finally dawned on me (and I am not proud to disclose this) that I was talking to an 83-year-old woman with an immune system compromised by 2 bouts of bladder cancer – a woman who suffered both pulmonary and coronary disease and who arrived at my office panting and leaning painfully on a cane. Despite these physical conditions, she was a formidable presence: A large forceful woman with a stentorian voice. But she knew full well that a cold could precipitate a hospitalization and lead to death. She had had a friend who had died that way. I had not tried to kill Frieda. But exposing her to my cold had indeed endangered her. Frieda was, admirably, doing everything in her power to survive, to fend off death. She had endured painful surgeries and highly unpleasant pharmacological treatments toward this end. And what had I done? I had invited the Grim Reaper into my office. In the end, I apologized. We agreed that in future if I had a cold, I would inform her, waive my cancellation policy and give her the choice about coming to my office.

This event happened years ago and alerted me to my need to do some homework. I had to ask myself why it had taken me so long to recognize the severity of Frieda's medical situation. I suspected that a part of the answer was to be found in a transference/countertransference dynamic, for pieces of Frieda's history had been played out in this interaction. Perhaps my lapse was an enactment in which my "role responsiveness" (Sandler, 1976) had led me to repeat the neglectful care Frieda had been subjected to in childhood. Or perhaps I had joined Frieda in her defensive denial of vulnerability. I also questioned whether I had, unawares, been acting out my own aggression toward Frieda – she had not been an easy patient. A recent battle over her demand that I call her doctors to scold them had left me bruised. But I had to be honest with myself. I sensed that there was more operating here and unless I understood my blindness, I was sure to repeat it with others. It was time for me to study myself. Finally, I recognized two difficulties that had interfered with my clinical functioning. First, I saw that despite my desire to provide my patient with an empathic, holding presence, I had been defending myself from feeling what it must be like to walk around the New York City streets or into a therapist's office with the knowledge that a cold can kill you. To resonate empathically with this degree of vulnerability would have been painful, and I had avoided that pain. Also, I had to acknowledge the extent of my denial of death, my failure to reckon with mortality. I had not faced that Frieda might die while in treatment with me. Or, although less likely, I could go first. These insights presented me with a homework assignment. To work well with older patients, I realized, I would have to grapple with the self-protective desire to shield myself from the degree of vulnerability and the proximity of death which my patients live with.

I have mulled over this incident, a mere half hour in the course of a long-ago treatment, for many years. I start with this because it portrays dramatically one of the transference–countertransference dynamics which may appear, usually with greater subtlety, in the work with many in Frieda's age group. In addition, it points to the need for those of us who treat older adults to do our "homework" – that is to come to know and to work with our feelings about aging, illness, and death.

Transference–countertransference patterns

The transference–countertransference configurations that arise in any treatment stem from a patient's unique relational history in interaction with the person of the therapist. They are specific to the therapeutic dyad. This is true of patients of all ages. Is there anything, one may then ask, distinctive about the transferences and countertransferences in work with the aged? Briefly, yes. With the understanding that each dyad is unique, a confluence of similar dynamics can result in commonalities, recurring patterns, to be found in these treatments. The therapist of the older patient can be helped by some familiarity with frequently recurring patterns.

Here I will discuss several patterns the therapist can look for including (1) transference and countertransference centered on the cast of characters of early relational trauma, (2) position in the life cycle of therapist and patient, and (3) extra-analytic transference. I will then turn to the emotional experiences of the analyst in reaction not to the dynamics of any particular patient but rather to old age and death themselves. I will close with a discussion of the therapist's homework: getting to know your personal equation.

Trauma: the original cast of characters revived

For those who were abused in childhood, we saw in Chapter 3, the ravages of older age can carry with them what Bromberg (2011) calls a tsunami, "the dissociated emotional disasters of early life that always seem to lie just around the corner" (p. 4). Long-dissociated self-states reemerge, bringing with them the affects and internalized relational patterns surrounding earlier trauma. It is as if the original childhood cast of characters from childhood come alive. These can inhabit the treatment room, expressing themselves in transference and countertransference. In a seminal work, Davies and Frawley (1994) explored the common transference–countertransference patterns that arise in the therapy of adults who have been sexually abused in childhood. While some of these patterns are specific to sexual abuse and thus include dynamics of seduction not necessarily present in other types of traumatic situations, the other patterns are often found with previously traumatized older adults, whether or not the trauma was sexual. The relevant transference–countertransference positions identified by Davies and Frawley are: (1) the unseeing, uninvolved parent and the unseen, neglected child, (2) the sadistic abuser and the helpless, impotently enraged victim, and (3) the idealized omnipotent rescuer and the entitled child.

Frieda, whom I endangered with my cold, exhibited all these versions of transference over time, while I had strong corresponding countertransference reactions. Early in the treatment she had experienced me as the rescuer – the caring parent she had yearned for – and she was my beloved child. When she clashed with her doctors and I refused to intervene, she experienced me as her passive father who had seen, yet tolerated, her abuse. Attempts I made to help her reduce her abrasiveness with medical personnel, hoping she would thereby receive better treatment, had been experienced as my collusion with the enemy. Then, when my behavior jeopardized her health, she experienced me as her abusive, neglectful mother – the mother who had beaten her, had humiliated her, and had refused to buy needed eyeglasses. My counter-transferences meanwhile ranged widely from highly pleasurable feelings of being a rescuer, to feelings of failure over my inability to save her, to guilt as a collusive bystander, and to shame that my contributions to her misery made me an abuser. When she screamed at me, she took on the role of the abusive mother, and I that of the abused, rageful, and powerless child. The very positions described by Davies and Frawley, the *dramatis personae* of Frieda's early trauma, were lived out with me.

Parents are supposed to keep their children safe. Likewise, analysts are supposed to keep their patients safe. An atmosphere of safety (Schafer, 1983) is considered essential to our work. When therapists speak of patient safety, they generally refer to psychological safety. Freedom from judgment, the permission to say what is socially proscribed, the certainty that no punishment will follow one's utterances, and confidentiality – these are the elements on which a therapeutic alliance can be built. The therapist's office should be a safe enough space that what is dangerous can be explored.

But what about physical safety? In most circumstances, analysts do not worry about that. The security both of the person and of the treatment setting are simply assumed. Until they are not. I still remember the ways my relationships with patients were transformed as we sat in my office during the World Trade Center attack. And Israeli therapists report the effect on therapy when patients and therapists were required to have gas masks at hand during sessions (Shoshani et al., 2010). Transference and countertransference are deeply affected when physical safety is in question. (I suspect that we still have much to learn about how they are affected by the risk of exposure to Covid-19.)

For the older patient, one component of safety is surely missing. We cannot keep our patients safe from disability, pain, and death. The rigors of older age evoke the need for an attachment figure who provides security. In this important respect, we fail. In trauma, the internal mother is allowing the attack to happen or at least failing to prevent it (Laub & Auerhahn, 1993). For patients who were not safe in their childhoods, this crime is a repetition. In the transference, this failure-to-protect makes us criminally negligent. I will continue the discussion of this topic, the therapist's failure to provide security in the face of death, in Chapter 6.

Position in the life cycle

Often the relative ages of analyst and patient have no bearing on transference. I have had patients twice my age who related to me as children, finding in me a parental presence. King (1980) described this phenomenon, saying "Patients may well experience themselves, in terms of psychological time-scale, as quite small and even helpless and the analyst as older" (p. 154). Reciprocally, I have felt a maternal countertransference, feeling their dependency and desiring to nurture them. Sometimes, however, transference and countertransference are in fact influenced by age difference.

Older patient, younger therapist

I first became aware of the way the transferences of older patients may be affected by their therapist's youth when, decades ago, I tried to understand why Hannah – a divorced woman in her 70s – kept changing her appointments. It gradually became clear to me that she was trying to be my last patient of the day. Was she trying to spend more time with me, I wondered? Was she eager to know what I was like outside the office or to establish a friendship? It was only when I learned that her 40-year-old unmarried son ferried her home from our appointments that I realized she wanted me to meet him. When I inquired about this, she confirmed my supposition. Her elaborate fantasy then emerged: I, a single woman at that time, would fall in love with her son, rescuing him from his lonely bachelor's existence and bringing a grandchild into her life. I joked with a colleague, borrowing from Gilbert and Sullivan, that in Hanna's transference, I was pegged as "daughter-in-law-elect," a position offered me by virtue of my age and single status. In the transference, Hannah was assigning me what Yalom (2008) calls an "immortality project" (p. 25). My producing a grandchild would grant her symbolic immortality via a biological mode (Lifton, 1979). Her fantasy was also an expression of generativity: I would be the recipient of what was most precious in her life, her son. And she would be giving her son something he lacked: a wife and a child.

Erotic transferences in older-patient-younger-therapist pairs may also present themselves, although ageist assumptions about loss of sexuality

may cause therapists to miss them. I finally recognized one in an octogenarian man when he told me how jealous his wife was at his spending so much
time with a pretty, younger woman. Mourning the loss of his sex life with
his now-disabled wife, in fantasy he made me the lover who kept his sexuality alive. His wife had sensed this dimension of his relatedness with me.

Sometimes, older patients assume the stance of parent or teacher to their
younger therapists. They will teach someone of relative youth either what
it is to be older or what they have learned in life. This stance may serve
multiple needs. It may be an attempt to "reverse roles" to compensate for
the humiliation of needing help. It may be an expression of generativity.
And for patients with either deep regrets or disappointments about their
parenting, this relationship may be experienced as an opportunity to finally
do a good job with a grateful child.

Dan, age 84, loved to tell me stories about his experiences in World War II.
I was fascinated by these and he knew it. A highly intelligent, observant
man, he was also able to reflect on the experience of aging and could tell
me what it was like to be an 84-year-old. Eventually his difficulties as a
parent emerged along with the pain he felt about his estrangement from his
son. He wished he had another chance as parent. In the transference, I was
the longed-for good child who would appreciate his efforts. I was already
familiar with my tendency to idealize patients (Schaffer, 2016). And I was
aware of Plotkin's (2000) warning about therapists' idealizations of older
patients. I had to work hard not to fall into a role of an adoring child – in
the process potentially losing sight of his difficulties.

In other cases, an older patient takes on a teaching role with a younger
therapist but may resent having to educate the therapist in order to be cared
for. Patients who were caretakers to their parents may be particularly sen-
sitive to this dynamic.

I was in my mid-40s. June, a long-divorced woman in her late 60s,
entered treatment because of a depression precipitated by the death of
her mother. Gradually her depression lifted and, as we explored other
issues in her life, I had the temerity to wonder whether seeking a roman-
tic relationship was one of her goals. June's response was to announce
her desire to leave therapy immediately. Fortunately, she was cooperative
with my request that we examine what was behind this desire. She was
then able to tell me that although she thought I was a good therapist who
had helped her, she felt that I did not understand what a woman her age
was up against in seeking romance or in deciding not to seek romance,

and she was sure that I would not be able to help her with that aspect of life. "How can you help?", she questioned. "At your age you don't have a clue. When I was your age, I didn't have a clue either." We then explored the meaning to her of my relative youth. I was non-defensive in acknowledging that I lacked the life experience she wished I had and that, therefore, there were aspects of her experience I did not understand. "I can imagine it's frustrating as hell to have to explain things to me which I would automatically know if we were the same age," I empathized. This exploration resulted in June's decision to stay in therapy. She then delved into the way my lack of knowledge about her world recalled the pain she had felt as a teenager when her immigrant parents had been unable to help her navigate the shoals of an American high school. Her anger at me had roots in the present and in the past.

Older therapist, older patient

Now that I am an older therapist, it is a pleasure to offer my older patients something I could not provide when younger: the experience of being understood by someone in the same boat. Older adults seek "the reassuring experience of essential alikeness" (Wada, 2003, p. 333). The twinship transference, Wada explains, fills self-object needs of elders at a time of severe narcissistic loss, fostering self-cohesion. Wada recommends therapist interventions that promote feelings of likeness. As an older therapist I can provide my older patient with the profoundly comforting feeling of likeness *sans* intervention!

   Sometimes, however, this similarity in ages can evoke negative feelings. Sibling transferences, too often neglected by analysts (Lesser, 1978), are not infrequent when therapist and patient are age-peers. Even without my disclosing much about my life, my patients know how I am weathering aging. They see that I am still working and earning an income, that I can get up from a chair without difficulty, and that my face does not bear the ravages of intense grief. A patient who concludes that I am not facing the tribulations that she faces may experience me as the favored child. Old issues about unfairness and jealousy emerge. The patient may experience shame over the feelings and have trouble verbalizing them. My countertransference may include a kind of survivor's guilt at life's bestowing preferential treatment on me. My countertransference may then cause me to collude in keeping those feelings out of the room.

Mary limps, leans on a cane, and uses a transportation service for the disabled to reach my office. We are about the same age. One day, she arrives early and sees me walking briskly down the street. She starts the session commenting on my gait and adds, "You must've done all the right stuff – exercising and eating and such – and now you're so healthy. I did all the wrong stuff and it's my own fault that I'm a physical wreck." I recognize Mary's pattern of turning aggression against the self and help her explore her feelings about our different health statuses. Shamefully, she confesses feelings of jealousy and resentment that my aging has been easier than hers. We also talk about the limitations of our control over our bodies' aging process. Mary then adds, "It's not fair that you can stride while I can only limp. It reminds me of how unfair it was that my sister was blonde and thin and I was neither. But, on the other hand, it's not fair that my brother is dead while I'm alive and that I can still go to the opera, which he loved. I guess life isn't fair, is it?" We grimace together and then laugh.

Even when therapist and patient are of similar ages, the patient may feel further along in the life cycle than her still-working therapist and may resent that. She may wish for a role model, to be led by someone "who has already been there." Dante had Virgil, who was already familiar with death, to lead him into the inferno. Our patients know we have not "been there." By virtue of our ability to work, we are demonstrating that we have yet to perform the labor of later old age. We are not yet the old old. Who are we to think we can help them face what we haven't yet faced ourselves?

Extra-analytic transference

With all patients, the exploration of transference is not limited to the analytic relationship; transference to others in the patient's life constitute a frequent source of insight. With older patients, in particular, this is the case. In Chapter 2, we examined the way relational configurations and conflicts from earlier developmental levels become alive in the ninth developmental stage. These may be writ large in the way patients perceive and relate to medical personnel, to dying spouses, to home-health aides, and to adult children. Patients' relationships with their bodies or body parts may also bear the stamp of early trauma. In these cases, mind and bodies are separated and an early object relationship may be played out between them. These patients may experience their suffering psyches as being at the mercy of their cruel, punishing bodies. Alternatively, they may punish their failing bodies by refusing to care for them, devaluing their bodies in the ways they were devalued as children. Much may be accomplished by working with this extra-analytic material in addition to the work focused on the therapeutic relationship. Carvalho (2008), for example, describes a case in which he focused almost exclusively on the relationship between the patient's mind and body, rather than on the transference to the analyst.

Susan's doctor knows the results of a scan revealing whether cancer has metastasized but does not return her phone calls. Harold is afraid to tell his financial advisor that his expenditures of the last quarter exceeded his predictions. Barbara's health aide rolls her eyes and sighs dramatically every time Barbara has an "accident." And Hazel's back punishes her every time she bends over. In each of these cases, my patient's reaction to the offending party will be influenced by early relational experiences. Much can be learned by an investigation of these relationships.

The analyst's emotional responses to the vicissitudes of old age

Colleagues and friends over the years, learning that I often work with older adults, have sometimes asked, "How can you do that? Isn't it depressing?" I answer that I find this work to be pleasurable and fulfilling; that I find it inspiring and life-affirming; that it is uniquely meaningful; and that it can touch me deeply. Some of my motivation for writing this book stems from my desire to counter ageist myths about the depleting nature of treatment of older adults. I hope that my case illustrations have conveyed my enthusiasm for this population and that I have given a taste of the joys to be gained. I would have left this field a long time ago if suffering were all!

It would be a mistake, though, to deny that practicing therapy with older adults can bring up less-than-pleasant feelings. Butler (1980) acknowledged this truth with his wry comment, "We psychiatrists are geniuses at understanding countertransference; surely we can recognize the ambivalence, dread, and concern we feel about aging, disability and death" (p. 10). Therapists working with this population should be prepared for such emotional experiences and should feel no shame about experiencing them.

Because older adults at times endure grievous physical and emotional pain, their empathic therapists may correspondingly suffer excruciating affects. That therapists treating trauma can be overwhelmed by harrowing feelings is now widely accepted. As Eshel (2016) put it, the unbearable experiences in working with traumatized patients can "permeate, attack and desecrate the analyst/therapist's psyche" (p. 98). The therapist of older patients knows all too well whereof she speaks.

My use of the term "excruciating affect" here is not hyperbole. Bucci (2018) teaches that there may be a neuropsychological basis to painful countertransference affects. Studies using functional magnetic resonance imaging and transcranial magnetic stimulation, according to Bucci, reveal that when someone observes another person's pain the same nerve cells fire as when he is in pain himself. Watching someone suffer causes suffering. Older patients can suffer tremendously; so, then, may their therapists. It is true that the older adult's therapist may not be exposed to the horror of immersing herself in the emotions of someone who has been tortured or raped. But there is a different kind of horror that can permeate this work. Therapists treating those facing the depredations accompanying older age know that they are getting a taste of what may well lie in store for themselves. They recognize the anguish that may lie ahead and they live with the reality of their mortality, whether they want to or not. They suffer.

It may, in fact, be the "suffering with," the co-suffering, which contributes to the therapeutic action. For the therapist cannot obliterate suffering. What we can do is "make suffering thinkable" (Berzoff, 2019, p. 119). Our deep emotional co-experiencing may be an important part of the therapeutic action. But make no mistake, the misery it involves can be truly miserable. It is important that we recognize our vicarious trauma and actively engage in self-care. I have found yoga, breathing exercises, talking to other therapists, and listening to music help. I encourage my fellow therapists to learn what works for them.

I believe that the therapist's processing of her traumatized reactions to her patient's trauma helps the patient. It is not, however, only the patient who benefits from this work. As we meet our patients' resilience in the face of trauma, we develop a "counter-resilience" (Gartner, 2014). We grow as well. As we face issues of mortality, the brevity of life, and how much of survival is mere luck, we mature. In helping our patients, we are helped as well on the long path of letting go of illusions of omnipotence, in treasuring life for what it is and mourning what it cannot be. We may endure pain in the process, but we also acquire a modicum of wisdom. Our patients are not the only ones who profit from this work!

The therapist's homework: getting to know your personal equation

Nineteenth-century astronomers, attempting the accurate measurement of heavenly bodies, learned that their measurements invariably disagreed with each other. Eventually, they realized that the observations of each individual astronomer differed from those of others in consistent ways. The term "personal equation" was then used to describe the consistent bias found in each astronomer's observations. Freud (1926) borrowed their term to describe the analogous effect that each analyst's personality has on what he or she perceives. Psychotherapists, like astronomers, have consistent biases. Our task is to learn our own.

To work with an older population, therapists must carefully examine their experiences of and attitudes toward aging, the aged, illness, loss, grief, and death. Let me add a plea here. I believe that our training programs, our training analyses, our peer supervision, and our study groups should be actively engaged with these issues. Existential issues require mutuality and containment. My discussions with other analysts lead me to believe that analytic training programs barely touch these issues. We must recognize a communal need to do more. Shapiro (2010) has made a similar suggestion. Noting that many beginning clinicians "have been fortunate enough to get through their personal analyses and their analytic training without any direct exposure to death" (p. 260), she recommends that training institutes teach about these issues. Charles (2015) reports on the vicarious trauma of caregivers to the traumatized and the ways support from others is ameliorative. Therapists are similarly affected by their immersion in the ordeals of their late-life patients and they, too, benefit greatly from group support. In my own work with older patients, I have consistently found this kind of support necessary and invaluable.

Therapists would do well to question what prejudices they have absorbed from our ageist society, prejudices that may influence their perceptions of the aged. One example of a common mistake by therapists working with older adults, springing from a societal stereotype of the aged as asexual beings, is a failure to inquire about the sex lives of their patients (Schwartz, 2019). It is also important to recognize the prejudices rampant in our profession. Yalom (1987) describes a predominant misconception of psychotherapy of older adults as, "a low throttle, low challenge variant of adult psychotherapy – a form of therapy which requires unusual patience and limited goals and is based on the belief that aged patients are disillusioned, demoralized [and] possess inelastic, resistive personality structures" (p. ix). This prejudice can lead a therapist to approach the treatment of older adults with low expectations rather than to recognize the potential for change. There are numerous studies which demonstrate that low expectations on the part of teachers strongly affect children's academic performance. Similar biases on the part of analysts may restrict a patient's potential growth. Or they may lead analysts into errors, such as attributing impairment of mental functioning to inevitable decline rather than looking for other causative factors, such as fear, depression, or over-medication (West, 2015).

It is important, too, that therapists examine the way their own histories, relational patterns, unfinished business with parents, and yearnings may influence their approach to older adults. Early experiences with aging, the aged and death should be explored. In addition, therapists' experiences subsequent to their own analyses may require self-analysis, to ensure an understanding of the way these experiences affect attitudes about aging. And, finally, therapists must wrestle with their own existential issues.

When I came upon Curtis's (2007) story about an incident in her analysis with the late Stephen Mitchell – a story painful to read in light of Mitchell's too-early death – I wondered if this was an example of an analyst's dodging issues of mortality. One day Curtis saw Mitchell jogging and, noting his flushed face, expressed concern about his health. Mitchell dismissed this quickly as an expression of her wish for his death. Mitchell, a pioneer in relational psychoanalysis and a consummate clinician, did not use this as an occasion for an exploration that could have been richly meaningful. Her feelings about loss and potential loss, her fantasies about his self-care, and her feelings about mortality – his and her own – much could have been revealed in such work. Of course, there may have been multiple reasons for Mitchell's response. Curtis's paper even offers at least one possibility: a much earlier dream in which she had hired the Mafia to kill her analyst. But Curtis in the moment had to correct Mitchell, to tell him that his flushed face had made her worry about his physical condition. Whatever the complex factors that contributed to Mitchell's clinical choice in this incident, it is not impossible – especially given our field's long abstention from dealing with existential issues – that he was under the sway of the same avoidance which had blinkered me when I exposed Frieda to my cold. To use Yalom's (2008) metaphor, he chose not to stare at the sun.

One final aspect of one's personal equation may need attention. I have posited (Schaffer, 2006) that the analyst's curative fantasies, which stem from childhood experiences and may have contributed to the choice of this profession, strongly affect clinical work. For therapists harboring these fantasies, the therapist's wishes to cure will be sorely tested in the treatment of older adults. Despite how much you can do, there is so much you cannot do to help the older patient. While your patient's mental health may improve considerably, you will have to watch her body decline, her losses accumulate, and, perhaps, her demise. Rescue fantasies will be activated and thwarted. To tolerate this process, grappling with these fantasies is part of the therapist's requisite homework.

References

Berzoff, J. (2019). Being still: Sitting with suffering in long-term relational practice. In S. A. Lord (Ed.), *Reflections on long term relational psychotherapy and psychoanalysis: Relational analysis interminable* (pp. 119–131). Routledge.

Bromberg, P. M. (2011). *The shadow of the tsunami and the growth of the relational mind.* Routledge.

Bucci, W. (2018). Emotional communication in the case of Antonio. *Psychoanalytic Inquiry, 38*(7), 518–529.

Butler, R. N. (1980). Research on aging: Its future in the United States. *The American Journal of Psychoanalysis, 40*(1), 3–11.

Carvalho, R. (2008). The final challenge: Ageing, dying, individuation. *The Journal of Analytic Psychology, 53*(1), 1–18.

Charles, M. (2015). Caring for the caregivers: Building resilience. *Psychoanalytic Inquiry, 35*(7), 682–695.

Curtis, R. C. (2007). On the death of Stephen Mitchell: An analysand's remembrance. In B. Willock, L. C. Bohm, & R. C. Curtis (Eds.), *On deaths and endings: Psychoanalysts' reflections on finality, transformations and new beginnings* (pp. 293–302). Routledge.

Davies, J. M., & Frawley, M. G. (1994). *Treating the adult survivor of childhood sexual abuse.* Basic Books.

Eshel, O. (2016). The "voice" of breakdown": On facing the unbearable traumatic experience in psychoanalytic work. *Contemporary Psychoanalysis, 52*(1), 76–110.

Freud, S. (1926). The question of lay analysis. In *The standard edition of the complete psychological work of Sigmund Freud* (Vol. 20, pp. 177–258). Hogarth Press.

Gartner, R. B. (2014). Trauma and countertrauma, resilience and counterresilience. *Contemporary psychoanalysis, 50*(4), 609–626.

King, P. H. (1980). The life cycle as indicated by the nature of the transference in the psychoanalysis of the middle-aged and elderly. *International Journal of Psychoanalysis, 61*, 153–160.

Laub, D., & Auerhahn, N. C. (1993). Knowing and not knowing massive psychic trauma: Forms of traumatic memory. *International Journal of Psychoanalysis, 74*, 287–302.

Lesser, R. M. (1978). Sibling transference and countertransference. *Journal of the American Academy of Psychoanalysis, 6*(1), 37–49.

Lifton, R. J. (1979). *The Broken connection.* Simon & Schuster.

Plotkin, F. (2000). Treatment of the older adult: The impact on the psychoanalyst. *Journal of the American Psychoanalytic Association, 48*(4), 1591–1616.

Sandler, J. (1976). Countertransference and role-responsiveness. *International Review of Psycho-Analysis, 3*, 43–47.

Schafer, R. (1983). *The analytic attitude.* Basic Books.

Schaffer, A. (2006). The analyst's curative fantasies: Implications for supervision and self-supervision. *Contemporary Psychoanalysis, 42*(3), 349–366.

Schaffer, A. (2016). The analyst's idealization of the patient: On not seeing the dark side. *Contemporary Psychoanalysis, 52*(4), 602–621.

Schwartz, K. M. (2019). Sexuality, intimacy, and group psychotherapy with older adults. *International Journal of Group Psychotherapy, 69*(1), 126–144.

Shapiro, S. (2010). Death in the consulting room: A review of *On deaths and endings. Contemporary Psychoanalysis, 46*(2), 258–268.

Shoshani, M., Shoshani, B., & Shinar, O. (2010). Fear and shame in an Israeli psychoanalyst and his patient: Lessons learned in times of war. *Psychoanalytic Dialogues, 20*(3), 285–307.

Wada, H. (2003). Chapter 15 The applicability of self psychology to psychotherapy with the elderly: With emphasis on twinship self object needs and empathy as a mode of observation. *Progress in Self Psychology, 19*, 331–343.

West, E. K. (2015). Being in time: The problem of hope in older adulthood, the last developmental frontier. *Issues in Psychoanalytic Psychology, 37*, 25–42.

Yalom, I. D. (1987). Foreword. In J. Sadavoy & M. Leszcz (Eds.), *Treating the elderly with psychotherapy* (pp. ix–xiii). International Universities Press.

Yalom, I. D. (2008). *Staring at the sun: Overcoming the terror of death.* Jossey-Bass.

Chapter 5

The narration of life stories and the self

I remember a square in Morocco piled with merchandise on rugs. Amid the heaps of clothing and spices, there were barbers cutting customers' hair, dental entrepreneurs with what looked like instruments of torture offering to pull teeth, and an old man on a chair surrounded by a large, rapt crowd telling a story. Humans love to hear stories. In addition, they compose their own every day. Most important are the stories they tell about themselves. The older adult has a long view back. A long life is seen as a whole and a story about this life can be told – to others or to the self. Self-narrative is an important component of an individual's identity and well-being. It is particularly important in older age when a summing up of one's life becomes a way of making meaning as one faces its ending.

In this chapter, I will first look at the value of self-narrative in later life and the importance of integrating relational and emotional meaning into the self-narrative. I will turn to the role that psychotherapy can play in promoting this integration and provide a clinical example. I will then turn to the forces that can sour or desiccate the self-narratives of later life and the work needed to counter them. I will end with the social narratives that unfortunately infiltrate the self-narratives of older adults.

The concept of self has a complicated history and definitions abound. Schafer (1992), noting this difficulty, states, "There is, I believe, some serious overloading of the conceptualization of self and possibly some theoretical incoherence as well" (p. 22). The term, however, is indispensable for understanding the experiences of older adults. I will be using the term in its experiential, subjective sense. With the recognition that there is multiplicity in self, that different self-states lead to different experiences of self at different times, I will be using it as it is used in common parlance, as when each of us asks the question, "Who am I?"

The functions of a life story

The sense of self, we saw in Chapter 3, can be battered by the traumatizing events of older age. Late-life trauma may shake the foundations of self
which are rooted in agency, in cohesion of the body, in connectedness to
one's past and future, and in one's affective life. Major losses, as we will
examine further in Chapter 7, can also radically alter the sense of self. The
construction of the self-narrative helps in the process of self-restoration.
It helps to knit together what feels fragmented, to reorganize a picture of
"who I am." As Köhler (2014) put it, "Autobiographical memory needs
the self, and the self needs autobiographical memory" (p. 19). The life
narrative not only restores and strengthens the sense of self, but it can also
foster a state of peace and of self-acceptance and help one face death. In
Charon's (2006, p. 178) words: "Many people with or without religious
affiliation who are facing death find the need to 'narrate' their experiences
as part of a search for meaning that in some way characterizes the essence
of the human condition." She is describing the ill, but these words are
equally apt for the old.

That older adults tend to look back and that they often recount episodes
from their earlier lives has long been recognized. Aristotle (1926), for
example, described the old as "continually talking about their past because
they enjoy remembering." At one time this reminiscing was viewed as
pathological, a way of escaping reality by living in the past, evidence of
encroaching senility. Butler (1963), a giant in the field of geriatric psychiatry who paved the way for much current work on mental health issues
in older age, however, viewed older adults' recalling their earlier lives
as constructive. Elders, he proposed, are not merely reminiscing but are
engaged in an active process of life review. This process, he explained,
can be used in the service of reorganization, of integration, and of the
reworking of unresolved conflicts. Butler's idea had a significant impact,
and the value of life review is now widely recognized – in fact, so widely,
that college students volunteering to work in nursing homes are taught to
facilitate it (Haber, 2006).

An intriguing view of the value of a self-narrative is offered by neurologists. As Siegel (2003) explains, to have a coherent story, the left hemisphere
must rely on information from the right. In healing trauma, he elaborates,
"neural integration can be achieved through the telling of coherent narratives" (p. 15). A similar view is held by Cozolino (2008), who states: "It is

my contention that social and private narratives support the growth, mutual activation and integration of diverse brain processes" (p. 194). Constructing a life narrative, they are telling us, is good for the brain!

DeYoung (2015), building on the work of the neurologists, states that to foster a coherent self, the self-narrative must be inclusive: It must integrate the recital of events provided by the left brain with the emotional and relational meanings provided by the right. "When the two sides of the brain aren't synchronized," she states, "the 'self' a person says he is can be quite different from the self he enacts in his emotions and relationships" (p. 104). This disjunction can be quite unsettling since the creator of narrative fails to understand the meanings or motivations surrounding the behavior being recounted.

In older age, the nature of one's self-narrative can make the difference between a state of misery or relative contentment. To reach that state of contentment, however, requires a narrative that is not merely a recital of events but rather a recital of events integrated with their emotional and relational meanings, as described by DeYoung. I suspect that the achievement of this kind of integration is what Erikson (1963) meant by his concept of "ego integrity."

The achievement of ego integrity requires, Erikson wrote, "the acceptance of one's one and only life cycle as something that had to be and that, by necessity, permitted of no substitutions" (p. 268). I was puzzled when I first read this. I asked myself why Erikson did not recognize that most common of feelings: regret. Surely, I thought, everyone knows that their life could have been lived differently. We say to ourselves, "If only I had chosen not to marry this person; if only I had accepted that job offer; if only I had listened to my parents; if only I had not listened to my parents." We know we made choices, sometimes poor ones. We regret, deeply and painfully. Over time, however, I have come to appreciate Erikson's insight: If we truly understand ourselves – our histories, internalized relationships, deep feelings, defenses, traumas, and pockets of pain – we realize that we had to do what we did. We may feel regret, but it is accompanied by self-understanding and self-acceptance. The events of our life are now integrated with their emotional and relational meanings. Our story is now enriched by our self-knowledge.

To get to this point, though, is often difficult and sometimes it cannot be reached on one's own. Psychodynamic treatment, in helping us understand what drove us, in reducing the volume of our self-persecuting inner voices, and in helping us understand and feel compassion toward the person we were when we made our choices, allows us to reach that place.

Psychodynamic psychotherapy and the self-narrative

One outcome of the psychodynamic psychotherapy of older adults is the amending and enriching of the patient's life story. As I'm doing the work, I may not be thinking of this as a goal. Together my patient and I are engaged in understanding her life and difficulties. We look for long-standing patterns, for hidden motivations, and for the parts of her experience she was forbidden or unable to know. We find words for what was previously unformulated (Stern, 1997). We trace modes of relating to the personalities and challenges met in early life. We examine the ways that she has learned to feel secure and investigate how these, while providing safety, may cause problems. And we use our relationship to explore old and new ways of being in the world. We don't just think together, we feel together. And we put into words the complex mix of feelings accompanying events – current and past – of the patient's life. In doing all this, we are co-creating the patient's story. Together we are generating a realistic self-narrative that does not omit disappointments and regrets but that weaves together good and bad. We are creating an integrated, complex, affectively rich tale. It is this work that leads to the outcome of the therapeutic process described by Cooper (2016), "the patient is able to hold the unsettling parts of his or her narrative in an easier position than before" (p. 30).

Gaining comfort with the unsettling parts of their narratives is especially important to older adults, for they know that the ends of their stories approach. Younger patients can compensate for an unsatisfactory past by imagining a dramatically different future. Older adults face that most of the story has already occurred and they must find a way to a self-acceptance which allows them to be at peace with the lives they have lived. The self-narrative that is imbued with self-understanding permits this.

Years ago, Katherine was abandoned by her bullying husband of 30 years. After she raised their five children, he had left her for a younger woman and, hiding his assets, succeeded in keeping alimony minimal. Katherine, facing her new challenges courageously, had started a small business selling art supplies, a business that had successfully met her modest needs. Now, retired, looking back on her life, she was tormented by self-reproach.

"I married him because I got pregnant," she told me. "When I realized what he was like, why didn't I leave him?" Answering that question, "Why didn't I leave him?" became one focus of our work. We had a clue when we began to see to what lengths Katherine would go to avoid my anger. Once, for example, she came to her session despite a very painful earache, because she was worried that canceling our appointment would get me angry. What would be the problem if I were angry? She would not only lose my good opinion, she told me, but she would also know that she was a bad person and would be filled with shame and self-loathing. Gradually a picture emerged. Katherine had identified with her bullied mother. She had learned to stay safe by appeasing her threatening father and whenever she experienced her own anger she worried that she was becoming like him. She had been intimidated by her ex-husband's anger and unaware of her own. In addition, her family and her priest would have condemned her if she left her marriage. She had wanted to keep her children secure. She had lacked the confidence that she could do what in fact she eventually did: find a way to manage on her own. As we fleshed out this picture, Katherine reached the place Erikson described: Hers was the only choice she could have made at that time. She wished her story could have been different and mourned what might have been. But she now had an autobiographical sense of self that she had never had before. Her life narrative had sadness etched in it; but it was imbued, too, with compassion for the self of her younger years who hadn't really had a choice. In the process of this work, too, she became less threatened by her own anger and less fearful of evoking the anger of others. These changes led to a new freedom in her relationships.

What makes a good story go bad?

Gaps in self-knowledge, we have seen, interfere with developing a coherent, integrated life narrative. In addition, there are other hindrances that may impede. I focus on three here. First, the memories available for the construction of self-narrative vary with mood and thus the self-narrative is susceptible to mood-related negative revision. Second, moral injury, the betrayal of one's own values, may be troubling enough to sour an entire narrative. And third, since a narrative always has a listener – internal or external – the relatedness with the listener can negatively affect the tone of the narrative.

Depression and the workings of memory

Memory researchers recognize a phenomenon they call "mood-congruent memory" (Watkins et al., 1996). Recall of earlier memories, they have discovered, is influenced by mood. One's current mood tends to facilitate the recall of memories that mirror it. This phenomenon may be related to the dissociative nature of the mind. As Bromberg (2011) notes, one's current self-state may lack access to memories of other self-states. The accessibility of memories is therefore in part a function of self-state. Perhaps this is why the retrieved earlier memories of depressed older adults often have a negative cast. A depressed state leads to the recall of depressing memories, omitting the good ones. In these cases, the self-told narrative, built on these negative memories, can become one of failure, self-loathing, and bitterness. Depression then evokes the recall of more negative memories that intensify the depression. If one of the tasks in older age is to make meaning of the arc of one's life, this task is undermined by these negative self-reinforcing cycles.

A visually arresting illustration of this phenomenon is found in a paper on narrative by Weisel-Barth (2019). She begins each case with a description of a patient's life of failure, ending that description with a statement such as, "This is Ella's story" (p 489). Then she switches to italics and, starting with the phrase *"Never mind that,"* she adds what the patient has omitted but has become known to the therapist – the many areas of the patient's life that were far from a failure, the hard-won accomplishments. The dramatic difference between the story told by the patient and the italicized story provided by the therapist brings home the "selective attention" (Sullivan, 1953) at work in the patient's construction of narrative. Depression facilitates the selection of depressing memories which make for a narrative of defeat – which reinforces the depression.

I became vividly aware of this issue when Shirley – painfully and with long pauses – told me her life's story of successive failures, including a disastrously disappointing career. I was extremely puzzled by this account because I was already acquainted with Shirley's story: She had been in therapy with me a decade and a half earlier. I already knew a lot about her life, minus the last 15 years, and the tale she was now telling bore little resemblance to the one I knew. True, Shirley's work life had had its disappointments. But what had happened to so drastically change her account? Shirley had been a pioneer in her vocation. As one of the first women hired in an all-male field, she had created innovative methods – methods still used today – for which she had never received compensation. However, those in the field knew of her major contributions and she had been highly regarded and admired by a large network of colleagues. Upon her retirement, coworkers had thrown a huge party to say goodbye to a valued colleague and to honor her creative contributions to the field. When we had last discussed her work life, she had been proud of her accomplishments, ruefully aware that her under-compensation was typical for women of her era, and able to enjoy the high esteem accorded her by those that mattered. Now, 15 years later, suffering a major depression, she remembered only her disappointments. "I was never promoted," she told me. "My career was a bust like everything else I've done."

Shirley's revision of her history after 15 years reveals the operation of "mood congruent" memory. In her depressed state, when she thought about her history, the negative memories were the ones she retrieved. Fortunately, as her mood improved, so did her self-narrative. Reflection on the changing view of herself was helpful, she told me. In the future, she would be more mindful of the way her fluctuating moods could cause her to rewrite history.

Moral injury

What if your narrative includes events where you betrayed your own values, where you harmed others? One aspect of the self-narrative in later life includes a moral reckoning. Partly emotional, partly cognitive, this reckoning gives an emotional cast to the story. It answers the question, "Have I been a good person?" This aspect of the self-narrative is compellingly present in the treatment of the military. Sherman (2014) describes veterans whose PTSD stems less from the violence of war and more from their guilt and shame over the part they played, or believe they played, in harming others. This "moral injury" can cause extreme psychic suffering and contributes, she tells us, to veterans' high rates of suicide. She describes the way a process she calls "self-empathy" can relieve, though perhaps not eliminate, this suffering. It is not rare for nonmilitary older adults, facing the ends of their lives and reviewing their life stories, to suffer similarly. That is, they recognize and feel a combination of guilt and shame about actions in their lives which have been damaging to others. And so troubling are these feelings, that they dominate the self-narrative.

Judy's daughter, Carol, struggles with substance abuse. While a skilled helping professional with many strengths, Carol has had long-standing financial and relational problems – at least in part caused by her addictive issues. Judy knows she drank during Carol's early years. "I never got drunk," she tells me "but I had a buzz most evenings, so I was tuning out a lot of what was going on. At some point, I realized this was harming her. I prayed a lot and went to AA meetings and have not touched alcohol since. But I'm sure my alcohol use is at the root of her problems. I hate myself for that."

How can a therapist help when older patients' distress is focused on moral injury – on the violation of their own moral codes, on the harm they have done others? The answer is a complex one, for this distress usually has multiple roots. At these times, in the face of a patient's self-loathing, I am frequently tempted to argue that the patient has done nothing wrong. I desperately want to soften my patient's self-punishment by declaring her innocent. To follow this impulse, however, would be a mistake. Judy knows that it would have been better for her daughter if she had used less alcohol during her early years; she and I must live with this painful reality. I cannot help by pretending this did not happen. Painful feelings must be lived through, not denied. Instead, my role is "compassionate witnessing." I need to help Judy face what she regrets, and to make this part of a much more complex story. Judy's current narrative is "I fucked up my kid. I'm bad." I need to help her write a less simplistic tale, one which does not villainize but also does not totally exonerate and one that does not deny the truth but that permits greater complexity and leaves room for self-compassion.

As we work in therapy, a multifaceted picture gradually takes shape. We come to understand the way Judy's history contributed to her drinking, the way her parents' histories contributed to their drinking, and the multiple functions this use of alcohol served. We examine the strengths that allowed Judy to stop when she did. We talk about the parts of her parenting of which she is proud, the way she searched the library for children's books related to her children's interests, her staying up all night to make them Halloween costumes. We do not omit the parts of parenting which she now regrets – not just the drinking but also the way she exposed her children to her rageful battles with her ex-husband. Judy tried very hard to be a good mother, but she coped with life's exigencies by utilizing the defenses she had developed in her own difficult childhood.

I tell Judy that I once saw a Superman movie in which Superman was able to spin the world backward in order to turn back time – and thus do what he had originally left undone. "Wouldn't it be wonderful," I mused aloud, "if we could turn back time based on what we know now." I am letting her know, without naming them, that I too have regrets. And together that we must mourn our lack of omniscience and omnipotence. In Sherman's (2014) discussion of moral injury of veterans, she noted the way that an assumption of omnipotence contributes to their suffering. They should have known, they omnipotently believe, that choosing to make that left turn would result in their buddy's death. To make one's regrets bearable, one must face that one is not, was not, omnipotent. Then the pain of regret may be lessened. But to let go of this faux omnipotence, we must mourn the vulnerability of the human condition. As we struggled with these issues, Judy became less self-punitive and less depressed. She mourned what she had been unable to do, recognized the good that she had done. Her life story had changed considerably.

To whom the story is told: relatedness to the listener

Constructing a narrative based on autobiographical memory is an interpersonal process (Stern, 2018). There is always a listener (even if an internal one) and the story is shaped by the state of relatedness with the listener. Therapists are the audience in the treatment room, and the narratives told will be affected by the patient's relatedness to the therapist. A patient may downplay accomplishments out of fear of evoking the therapist's envy. A sad narrative may be offered in a bid for nurturance, perceived as available only to sufferers. Or it may be a veiled accusation: "Look at my misery. You haven't helped me." A triumphant tale may be told, not because it feels true to the patient but in an attempt to meet the therapist's narcissistic needs.

Ivan knows that I am writing about him, since I have asked his permission to include his (disguised) case material in a paper. Now he is in distress when he faces telling me about a new problem. He apologizes profusely. As we try to understand this, it becomes clear that he feels driven to perform well. He must present a perfect life, so that I can feel like a good therapist/writer and tell a story of a successful treatment. We see an old pattern: Ivan is trying to take care of me in the same way he took care of his mother. He never complained to her about his father's violence because his unhappiness made her feel like a bad mother. There may, however, be more to this. Ivan accurately recognizes that I bring narcissistic needs to my writing. Have I sent him the message that I need him to remain trouble free, that I want a happy ending to his story? Our recognition of these currents is important. Ivan will lose the benefits of creating an integrated, meaningful life narrative if he persists in creating two stories: a triumphant one for me and a sadder one he holds within.

As older adults sum up their lives to search for meaning, it is not rare that a long-dead parent becomes chief listener and critic. When this occurs an internalized voice of the past, now revived, may cast shadows on one's life narrative. Even people who seem well "individuated," having followed their own paths rather than those prescribed by their parents, can be brought up short by the recognition that it is now too late to satisfy the wishes of (long-deceased, internalized) parents. And that it is too late to win their approval. The arc of a life, now viewed as if through parental eyes, spells failure. Separating and individuating, becoming one's own person, are often viewed as occurring in one's early years. But this process continues through the life span (Colarusso, 2000). In older age, creating a good narrative may require another foray into this process. To shed feelings of failure, one may once again have to face the discrepancy between the life led and the life one was supposed to lead. There is mourning involved. One has been graced with only one life and it may have been insufficient to accomplish one's multiple conflicting goals.

Brian, in his 60s, feels like a failure because he lives simply, with few material possessions. Despite his parents' goals for him, he had dropped out of law school and instead made a life in the arts. It was a creative life and one he relished, but it was poorly remunerated. One day, he is pouring out evidence of his shortcomings, telling me that he owns no house, no car, and no "good watch." I ask, "And those are things you have always wanted for yourself?" He is flummoxed, pauses, and then grins. "No," he tells me, "those are the things my parents wanted for me. I'm a Bohemian. I've always been happy living in a garret and buying my clothes in thrift shops." The origins of his depression are now much clearer. We have much to work with.

Sometimes, the culprit behind a life narrative of tragic failure is an internal torturer. This inner critic can cause regrets to become overpowering and one's narrative a story of a wasted life. The presence of an internal persecutor may explain one of the findings of memory researchers. In depressed states, people tend to exaggerate their agency regarding negative events and downplay it for their achievements (Habermas, 2015). Their harsh self-evaluators attribute their successes to luck and their failures to their own stupidity. Usually the persecutory internal voice is not a newcomer, but it may become over active in later life. The older adult has to face that this is the life she has lived, with whatever disappointment it contains, and that there is no "redo." Because the future is now foreshortened, fantasized future accomplishments can no longer be used to appease the inner tormenter. This may require mourning and "coming to terms with" – processes greatly hindered by self-condemnation. Methods for self-restoration that one has used in the past, such as proving one's worth to oneself by manic productivity, may no longer be available. However, psychotherapeutic work, by softening the condemnation of the persecutor, may help.

Susan had always attacked herself mercilessly. She had long thought this style of self-relating was a good thing: after all it drove her to do her best. But now, postretirement, she recognizes that it prevents her from feeling satisfied with the life she has lived. Together we learn to recognize when this persecutor is activated. We call it "Pete," recognizing it as the voice of Susan's deceased but internalized critical father. We "talk back" to it. We even make fun of it: "There he goes again." Psychotherapy does not destroy Susan's internal persecutor. It does, however, make it easier to live with.

Social narratives

It is not only individuals who have stories. Our society embraces stories as well, stories that embody shared values, and which deeply infiltrate their members' self-perceptions. Four of these, in particular, do damage to older adults and contribute to soured life narratives. Therapists should be aware of these stories and their effects on older adults. I have found that calling attention to them and discussing them with patients reduce their power.

Rugged individualism and self-reliance

With its foundational stories of pioneers leaving their countries of origin and striking out into wilderness, the culture of the United States has long esteemed self-reliance and the courageous overcoming of danger. The self-made man who needs nobody and has total responsibility for the life he creates has long been our hero. We honor the cowboy who can face and defeat enormous odds and then ride off into the sunset alone.

The value system entailed in this cultural icon is alive and well in our current socioeconomic system. A neoliberal approach (enormously profitable to certain members of our society) sends the message that individuals are totally responsible for their own positions in life. Poverty is the fault of the individual. Educating your child is your responsibility and if you are unable to provide a college education, you have handled your finances irresponsibly. Paying for medical care is your responsibility even when the price of your medication skyrockets. Society should not supply what self-reliant individuals should be supplying for themselves. In this view, older adults should be able to pay for basic needs, such as dentistry, hearing aids, eyeglasses, and, if needed, long-term care. If they cannot, they've mismanaged their lives.

Repeatedly, I have found that this story line infects the self-narrative of older adults. Not being able to manage what is unmanageable and not having the resources requisite for some degree of comfort in later life when the demand for such resources is unreasonable – these troubles are often not recognized as resulting from problematic aspects of our society rather than individual failure.

After a lifetime of work as a civil servant, Janet has carefully planned her retirement budget and has found ways to stay comfortable while remaining frugal. Suddenly, she is "short." What has happened? The price of her diabetes medication tripled, her medical insurer refused to reimburse her for the outpatient surgery her physician had recommended, and an abscessed tooth recently required expensive dental work. She is able to pay her rent now only by borrowing money from her brother, an act she finds humiliating. The life story she now tells herself is one of inadequacy and defectiveness.

The guilty party is mother

A second social narrative, unfortunately once fostered by psychoanalysts, places the responsibility for a child's emotional problems squarely on the mother. The most egregious instances of this lay in attributing childhood autism to "the refrigerator mother" and psychosis to the "schizophreno-genic mother." Although, these attributions are now outmoded, the narrative persists that good parenting results in problem-free children and that an adult child's difficulties represent a mother's failure. Many older women, therefore, suffer greatly when their adult children struggle. It is hard enough to face old age and death and realize you will no longer be there to help your children, to protect them, and to comfort them. But it is doubly hard when you excoriate yourself, believing that you are the cause of all their problems. Older mothers often have regrets about how they handled aspects of parenting. And, of course, problematic parenting does in fact contribute to a child's difficulties. Older adults, we saw, suffer moral injury when they recognize and regret harm they have done their children. But to adhere to the sense of a failed life because your adult child's life is not running smoothly is to incorporate the social narrative, "blame the mother."

Sharon, age 74, is deeply involved with her 44-year-old single daughter's pain over never having married. She recognizes that her daughter has had difficulty in her relationships with men and believes, not without reason, that this difficulty stems from her relationship with her hypercritical father, the ex-husband Sharon chose to marry at the age of 21. Sharon therefore blames herself for her daughter's distress – her early marital choice harmed her beloved child. Sharon's self-blame leads to a life story revolving around her failures as a mother. This life story contributes to her depression, a depression that then adds to the negative shading of her life story. Part of Sharon's problem may stem from her "internal persecutor" – an attacking part of herself which leads her into self-blame. But her internal prosecutor is considerably strengthened by the social myth that mother is always at fault: if her daughter has problems, she was a bad mother.

The strong triumph over nature; only the weak succumb

In our society, we share the illusion that if we just fight hard enough, we can triumph over cancer and we can defeat death. We are pitted against nature, and there is barely a wisp of recognition, not to mention acceptance, of the limits of our control. Even when the worst happens, we are supposed to face this with heroism, optimism, and courage – fighting to the end. To succumb to nature is to lose a battle and to feel weak or vulnerable is to fail.

Cancer survivors speak openly about the pressures they feel to prevail in battle. Their relatives want to be able to report in obituaries, "She bravely fought." Military metaphors abound and there is no room for the story, "She suffered a lot and had a hard time of it. Eventually it killed her and we're sorry she had to suffer so." Notable among these survivors is the psychoanalyst Kathlyn Conway (2007), who tells us, "By subscribing so insistently to the narrative of triumph, we participate in a hysterical denial, as if by chanting 'triumph' we can ward of mortality" (p. 18). The social narrative of triumph, Conway says, blinds us to the survivor's actual experience of fragility, of destabilization of the self, and of pessimism or outright despair. Commenting on Oliver Sacks' treatment by a surgeon who insisted on a narrative of triumph, she notes that the doctor's refusal to hear Sacks' "less triumphant story" led his patient to serious psychological difficulty. Similarly, the discrepancy between older patients' increasing fragility and the social narrative of triumph over nature leads to profound experiences of not being seen and to the self-experience of failure.

"What's wrong with me that I don't want to fight?" says Joan. "I want a peaceful end to my life. But the nurses keep telling me I should fight harder. Why am I such a wuss?"

Older adults are "Past it"

Corporations have learned the hard way that "engineering and promoting new products and services especially designed for the expanding market of the aged is a good way of going out of business" (Gopnik, 2019, p. 37). Gopnik reports on numerous entrepreneurial ventures that appear brilliant in their recognition of the needs of older adults and in their innovative solutions to these needs – all of which have failed or performed abysmally. His conclusion should give us pause, "We would rather suffer because we're old than accept that we're old and suffer less" (p. 37). Perhaps we should rephrase his conclusion: We would rather suffer because we're old than endure the even worse suffering we would endure if we were to take on the devalued identity of being aged. As Gopnik says, "identity matters to us far more than utility" (p. 37). And in an ageist society, nobody wants to identify as old. Through the lens of ageism, older adults in Western society are viewed as ugly, depressed, senile, passive, weak, cranky, or boring. This is the story these negative stereotypes tell: Whoever you were before, in your final years you have little to offer.

Older adults receive the messages about who they are from the way others treat them. When people talk down to them as if they have minimal intelligence, when people in their presence talk about them as if they are not there, when people assume that they are incapable and uninteresting, and when people shunt them off to settings invisible to the rest of society, older adults absorb negative portraits-of-self. In addition, as members of our ageist society, they have internalized these same negative stereotypes. As a result, the narratives of older adults may have unduly sad endings: Once I was something, now I'm worthless.

The effects on older adults of their own negative stereotypes are now being studied, with dramatic findings. Research provides evidence that older adults' ageist beliefs are powerful enough to interfere not only with the sense of self but even with physical functioning. I am particularly intrigued by an ingenious study performed by Becca Levy and others (Levy et al., 2014). Recognizing that it is difficult to change internalized stereotypes because individuals' cognitive processes often work to preserve existing beliefs, these researchers sought a way to bypass consciousness, to affect older adults' beliefs implicitly. (You could say they wanted to speak directly to the unconscious.) To accomplish this, they exposed their sample of older adults (mean age 81) to subliminally presented visual cues – that is, to visual stimuli presented so briefly that they were a blur. The participants could not say what they had seen; the stimuli were not consciously registered. To counter their internalized negative beliefs about aging, the experimental group were exposed to visual stimuli containing positive statements about aging over a period of weeks, and the results were dramatic. These people performed significantly better than a control group (exposed similarly to neutral stimuli) on measures of physical functioning, such as time to rise from a chair or to walk eight feet. This experiment demonstrates the profound effect of ageism on the aged. It also demonstrates the potential effect of countering ageistic beliefs, of instilling a different social narrative about what it is to grow old. Psychotherapists can take heart from this study: our older patients may benefit greatly if our work succeeds in transforming their internalized beliefs about aging.

For some older individuals, membership in a stigmatized group is a first-time occurrence. While they may retain a degree of privilege, they are now forced to confront their lowered status. For others who are already members of groups subjected to discrimination, the insults of being seen as inferior add to previous injuries. I believe that there is more we need to learn about intersectionality with respect to aging. The stories individuals tell about themselves will be influenced by the "isms" to which they are, and have been, subjected.

We all lose out when the narratives of the older members of our society are not valued, for the stories that elders tell are of benefit not merely to themselves but also to others. Lipton (2019) describes her father's story-telling, with its ever-changing details of the ways he overcame hardships, as not only a way to process his own earlier trauma but also to foster resilience in younger family members. The stories of elders, if anyone listens, may be a generative gift to future generations. But in an ageist society few may listen.

References

Aristotle. (1926). *Aristotle in 23 Volumes* (J. H. Freese, Trans.). Harvard University Press.

Bromberg, P. M. (2011). *The shadow of the tsunami and the growth of the relational mind.* Routledge.

Butler, R. (1963). The life review: An interpretation of reminiscence in the aged. *Psychiatry, 26*, 65–76.

Charon, R. (2006). *Narrative medicine: Honoring stories of illness.* Oxford University Press.

Colarusso, C. A. (2000). Separation-individuation phenomena in adulthood: General concepts and the fifth individuation. *Journal of the American Psychoanalytic Association, 48*(4), 1467–1489.

Conway, K. (2007). *Illness and the limits of expression.* University of Michigan Press.

Cooper, S. H. (2016). *The analyst's experience of the depressive position: The melancholic errand of psychoanalysis.* Routledge.

Cozolino, L. (2008). *The healthy aging brain: Sustaining attachment, attaining wisdom.* W.W. Norton.

DeYoung, P. A. (2015). *Understanding and treating chronic shame: A relational neurobiological approach.* Routledge.

Erikson, E. H. (1963). *Childhood and society* (2nd ed.). W.W. Norton.

Gopnik, A. (2019, May 20). Younger longer: Can the infirmities of aging be postponed. *The New Yorker*, pp. 36–43.

Haber, D. (2006). Life review: Implementation, theory, research and therapy. *International Journal of Aging and Human Development, 63*(2), 153–171.

Habermas, T. (2015). A model of pathological distortions of autobiographical memory narratives: An emotion narrative view. In L. A. Watson & D. Berntsen (Eds.), *Clinical perspectives on autobiographical memory* (pp. 267–290). Cambridge University Press.

Köhler, L. (2014). On the development of the autobiographical self and autobiographical memory – Implicit and explicit aspects. *International Journal of Psychoanalytic Self Psychology, 9*(1), 18–34.

Levy, B. R., Pilver, C., Chung, P. H., & Slade, M. D. (2014). Subliminal strengthening: Improving elders' physical function over time through an implicit-age-stereotype intervention. *Psychological Science, 25*(12), 2127–2135.

Lipton, J. (2019). Constructing trauma's narratives in the later years: Aging and the life review. *Contemporary Psychoanalysis, 55*(3), 147–163.

Schafer, R. (1992). *Retelling a life: Narration and dialogue in psychoanalysis.* Basic Books.

Sherman, N. (2014). Recovering lost goodness: Shame, guilt, and self-empathy. *Psychoanalytic Psychology, 31*(2), 217–235.

Siegel, D. J. (2003). An interpersonal neurobiology of psychotherapy: The developing mind and the resolution of trauma. In M. F. Solomon & D. J. Siegel (Eds.), *Healing trauma: Attachment, mind, body and brain* (pp. 1–56). W.W. Norton.

Stern, D. B. (1997). *Unformulated experience: From dissociation to imagination in psychoanalysis*. Analytic Press.

Stern, D. B. (2018). How does history become accessible? Reconstruction as an emergent product of the interpersonal field. *Journal of the American Psychoanalytic Association, 66*(3), 493–506.

Sullivan, H. S. (1953). *The interpersonal theory of psychiatry*. W.W. Norton.

Watkins, P., Vache, K., Verney, S., Muller, S., & Mathews, A. (1996). Unconscious mood-congruent memory bias in depression. *Journal of Abnormal Psychology, 105*, 34–41.

Weisel-Barth, J. (2019). Stories that open and stories that close: Theoretical and clinical narratives in psychoanalysis. *Psychoanalytic Inquiry, 39*(7), 485–493.

Chapter 6

Existential anxieties

One morning, as Gregor Samsa was waking up from anxious dreams, he discovered that in bed he had been changed into a monstrous verminous bug.

Kafka, the genius who wrote that sentence, never had the good fortune to grow old. He experienced the dehumanization for which Gregor's tale serves as metaphor in other spheres of life. It is uncanny, therefore, to what extent *Metamorphosis* aptly depicts old age in its most nightmarish version. This is the old age nobody wants.

Gregor wakes up having to face that he is an animal. He has turned into something loathsome both to himself and to others. He can no longer control his body and formerly effortless movements now cause pain. He lives in constant terror of falling. He feels shame about his ugliness and does his best to hide it. He can no longer provide for others and instead, disgracefully, needs care. He is shunted aside, isolated from the community he used to belong to. The care he receives is wretched. He longs for a mother. Others no longer understand his communications. Others see him as monstrous, as no longer human. Eventually, he is dead and thrown out in the trash. And then he receives the final narcissistic blow – after he is gone, others thrive.

Older adults may live that nightmare. They are forced to recognize that they are no more than animals and that they are, in Becker's (1973) words, "housed in a heart-pumping, breath-gasping body that once belonged to a fish and still carries the gill-marks to prove it" (p. 26). They must reckon with unwelcome changes to and the loss of control of their bodies. They may experience feelings of repulsiveness, social exclusion, and humiliating dependency. Hit with the sorry truth that death approaches, that it cannot be stopped, and that life will go on without them, they may end up feeling like Gregor: less than human, disposable, and worthless. They may believe that their lives have no meaning and that all they can hope for are weary existences bereft of value or pleasure as they await the end. And that then, like Gregor, they will be discarded.

Isn't it interesting that among the symptoms so neatly categorized in the DSM V's (American Psychiatric Association, 2013) immense compendium of psychological woes, one has been left out: existential anguish? Perhaps the anxiety, emptiness, and despair that may come from recognizing one will die and the profound worry that one's life has had no meaning do not constitute a mental disorder. But existential pain qualifies as one of the most tormenting of psychic aches. In addition, existential torment may well fuel many of the symptoms DSM does recognize. In older adults, while survival concerns, physical pain, and other reality challenges may force attention away from these issues, in the background they lurk. As humans face their finitude, they wonder: "Must I really die?" "Is there no way to stop that?" "How do I bear it?" "What has this been about?" "Has my life meant anything?"

I am going to discuss three existential tasks that may overwhelm and bring distress in older age. In each case, I will focus on the nature of the task and on how therapists can facilitate their patients' work on it. In each case, this work may promote growth. The first task is the transition of the prospect of death from an intellectual concept to a felt experience. Next is the search for meaning. Finally, there is the process of reckoning with one's lack of omnipotence and of finding a way to surrender to the inevitable while retaining agency. Since these tasks are requisite for all humans, therapists face them as well and – if they are honest with themselves – they know their own struggles with them. Fortunately, one need not have mastery of a task to help others with it. In fact, therapists may find that their work with patients on these issues helps them in their own existential work.

The transition to death as a felt experience

"Lucky the leaf unable to predict the fall," wrote Auden. Unlucky are humans: We predict the fall. Often our awareness of death remains intellectual. Through much of our lives we know that someday we will die, but we may not feel it. In older age, death becomes less abstract. Older adults – besieged as they are by the losses of age-peers, by their own "health scares," and by watching the rise of their chronological ages – may reside in what Brody (2016) calls "night country." The prospect of death becomes all too real. Some face the reality of death and are overwhelmed. Others look away. Either of these reactions may be problematic.

The difficulty of the older adult who is overwhelmed by facing death is often apparent, for being flooded by terror may precipitate symptoms, such as an agitated depression or substance abuse. Less visible may be the difficulties inherent in the flight from the recognition of mortality – a flight encouraged by the norms of our ageist, youth-oriented society. Alpert (2012) describes the trouble caused when the chronically ill try to "pass" as healthy. In participating in the "theater of pretending" (p. 129), she warns, it may seem true that you can hold onto the healthy self you have been most of your life, but the price of passing may be that the disavowal of central parts of your own experience can lead to feeling "dead, disconnected, detached, and inauthentic" (p. 119). Elders who flee knowledge of their progression through the life span may pay the same price. Sometimes it may seem worth paying that price to avoid the destabilization that may attend the recognition of one's finitude. To be fully alive in older age, however, one must connect affectively with one's experiences of moving toward life's end while embracing the life one has.

This undertaking is captured in Shakespeare's 73rd sonnet. Shakespeare gives words to the poignant losses and decrepitude of older age: "Bare ruin'd choirs, where late the sweet bird sang." Then he ends the sonnet: "To love that well which thou must leave ere long." That is what we hope for – for ourselves and our patients. We want to acknowledge the "bare ruin'd choirs," to face our losses and our impermanence and yet to love the people and the life we must leave "ere long." How can psychotherapists help?

Most important, we provide a place to reflect and talk about these issues. People do better when they do not face them in isolation and silently. Yet we live in a society that discourages talking about the end of life. For many older adults, simply the opportunity to talk with someone who can bear to hear, who can remain emotionally present while hearing, is valuable. Any number of patients have said to me, "I think about this a lot, but I have never talked to anyone about it before." And talk we do. In fact, one of the ways the therapy of seniors differs from that of younger patients is that existential issues arise more often and, when given voice, add depth and urgency to the work. In doing so, we join our patients, bearing the powerful feelings that facing mortality evokes, providing the "sustained relational engagement" that Frommer (2005, p. 555) identifies as requisite.

There may be times we need to clear away the obstacles that prevent patients from speaking of existential issues. They may, for example, worry about depressing the therapist, especially if their parents were intolerant of the expression of negative affect. They may fear the judgment that they are "morbid." Or they may worry that talking about death makes it more likely. Analyzing the difficulties that make discussing these topics threatening allows them into the room and fruitful work can follow. Therapists learn about their patients' feelings and fears, their early encounters with death, and their images and fantasies of their own deaths. Simply talking about these issues makes them less toxic. Unformulated and unexpressed, these fears may have a life-constricting grip. Exposed to the open air, they may become part of a more fully vitalized life – a difficult part, it is true, but only a part.

To talk the talk, one must walk the walk. Perhaps in treating 20-year-olds one has the luxury of intellectual conversations about death. When one is speaking with a septuagenarian or octogenarian, however, the need is for more than that. One is not helping if one presents with what Cooper (2016) names "postured equanimity" (p. 43), simulating the acceptance of limits. To talk meaningfully about death, one must oneself face feelings of impermanence. According to Symington (2006), "If in an engaged relationship between two people one of the two has faced the fear of death, then the other person has a good chance of being able to do so also" (p. 72). I have, indeed, faced the fear of death; but every time I have done so, I have successfully unfaced it soon afterward. Yalom (2008) would understand, as he equates facing death with staring at the sun: You can't do it for long. In talking about death with my older patients, I strive to keep my impermanence a felt experience. Sometimes I succeed and sometimes I don't. Perhaps the trying is, in itself, helpful. For my patient and I are joined in our mutual vulnerability, including sharing the experience of trying to digest the indigestible, the fact that we will die.

Treating early trauma is another way we help patients when their fears of death overwhelm. Death terrifies, but it may be that much more terrifying to those who suffered early trauma. Clement (2005) provides an example. Her patient participated in a meditation retreat focused on death and the experience plunged her into a destabilizing episode of grief and despair because, it emerged in her analysis, it brought up powerful feelings of early trauma. The felt experience of death, I have learned, is a trigger, reviving earlier experiences of suffering while helpless. These may cloak fantasies of death with aspects of early trauma. The containing function of the therapist can render the traumatic affects bearable enough that they can be thought about and talked about. Links between early experiences and envisioned death are then apparent. Working with the early trauma in these cases, does not remove the fear of death, but it may diminish its horror. Claire, we saw in Chapter 2, was helped when we recognized that she fantasized death as a repetition of her early experience of being sent away to boarding school.

Anna, whose story is told in Chapter 7, is another example of someone whose early trauma intruded into her felt experience of the approach of death. Hers was a premature birth and she spent her early months first in an incubator, then isolated in a hospital. Now, in her late 80s, she wasn't especially frightened of death itself, she told me, but she was terrified of being buried alive. That she didn't trust the competence of doctors and undertakers was clear. But there was more here. We came to understand this after an upsetting incident in which she fell in her bathroom, could not get up or yell loudly enough to be heard by her husband, and lay covered with feces all night. We talked out in detail what that had felt like. And as we did that, we realized that the experience – awful in its own right – might also have revived early preverbal, sensory memories of her months as an infant in an incubator and a hospital. Could this also help explain her terror of waking up in a coffin covered with dirt with no one there to hear her scream? I told Anna about Winnicott's theory that the breakdown feared is the one that has already happened. I wondered if the death she feared was the experience that had already happened, being enclosed in an incubator with nobody responding to her cries. We discussed this possibility and together we put into words what the tiny infant Anna must have felt in that incubator. The Anna of today wished she could have uttered comforting, soothing words to her younger traumatized self. Together, we murmured them. Since we did this work, she reports that she is still afraid of dying but is no longer preoccupied by the fear of being buried alive.

The search for meaning

Humans engage in "never-ending efforts at building good-enough meanings in face of a haunting, background awareness of our allotted speck of time, on a speck of a planet, in an infinite universe" wrote Slavin (2016, p. 542). These efforts become more urgent as one's allotted speck of time on this speck of a planet draws to an end. In facing death, we search for meaning. That is one of the essential tasks of older age. Can the therapist help? To facilitate a search for meaning is a tall order, for the task has spiritual, religious, and philosophical as well as psychological dimensions. Does it even make sense to take this on? Lev (2016) answers this question in the affirmative, observing a movement in psychoanalysis toward the spiritual. But our training has not prepared us for this. How do we help our patients in the search for meaning?

Fortunately, we need not answer that question in the abstract. One of the striking things about facilitating quests for meaning is that patients lead the way. At times their distress is extreme enough that emotional survival, not the search for meaning, is paramount. And then, as suffering becomes manageable, I watch them seek to participate in their lives in ways expressive of who they are, which embody their values, which provide them with a sense that their lives matter. "Engagement," says Yalom (1980) is the therapeutic answer to meaninglessness" (p. 482). What I have learned is that meaning comes not by soul-searching and not by grand gestures but rather by the texture of one's participation in daily life. My patients find meaning in the ways they live their lives.

For some, self-expression in the arts provides the sense of meaning. Eliot, whose story is told in Chapter 3, was one of those.

For some, recognition of their participation in the web of life does the same. I remember a phone session interrupted when my patient, looking out her window, saw an eagle being mobbed by smaller birds. "They are protecting a nest," she told me. "Isn't it amazing, what animals will do to keep each other safe. I guess I'm doing the same thing when I give my granddaughter her vitamins." I could tell she was beaming.

For some, meaning is found via religious belief. Patients may bring to therapy obstacles that interfere with their finding comfort in their faith. "I'll tell you what frightens me about dying," says Patricia, a Roman Catholic woman in her 70s. "When I taught at a community college, 17-year-old freshman girls would come to me, suicidal because they were pregnant. I told them where they could get advice about abortion. You know I am totally opposed to abortion, that I believe it is murder. And yet I did that. When I stand before God, He will see me as a murderer." I listen and feel for Patricia. What can I, proudly pro-choice, say to help? I suppose I can don my psychoanalytic hat and note the way her picture of God shares her father's judgmental qualities. I suppose I can explore her wish that I have the priest-like power to absolve her of sin. Or I could identify this as a religious issue to be discussed with a priest. Instead, I say, "It is hard for me to believe that a loving God would judge so harshly an act done out of compassion." She nods, thoughtful.

Who am I to be talking about what happens after death and about the nature of God? This is one of many instances where I find myself dipping into spiritual issues, simply because they are alive in the room. These come up often and even as I feel out of my depth, I welcome them. For I know my patient is doing important work and that I am privileged to be part of this conversation. I must remind myself that I need not have the answers: I simply need to be part of the conversation.

Many older adults use the mode Solomon et al. (2015) have studied, finding ways to feel like "a valuable contributor to a meaningful world" (p. 60). One of my patients endures significant physical discomfort weekly to attend a prayer circle devoted to prayer for immigrants, for the climate, and for world peace. Another takes periodic bus rides to Albany to meet with New York State legislators about issues meaningful to her. Both describe these experiences as giving them a sense that their lives are worthwhile.

And many patients find meaning by a route Lifton (1979) describes as, "the humble everyday offerings of nurturing or kindness in relationships of love, friendship, and at times even anonymous encounter" (p. 22). In their thirst to engage with others in ways that afford meaning, patients make concerted efforts in their therapy to work through conflicts inhibiting self-expression and intimacy. The therapist assists by recognizing the urgency and significance of their quest.

Jill, ashamed about her drinking when her son was young, discovers he now has a "drinking problem." Guilty and terrified, she becomes judgmental, lecturing him on the evils of alcohol. The two exchange tense words. "I wanted to help him," she told me, "but I made things worse. Now he's mad at me. Maybe, if I wait a couple of months, he'll have forgotten it and we can go back to normal. What should I do?" I suggest we talk about it more. She works then on her painful regrets and on the shame she still experiences about her drinking. She expresses the wish she knew then what she knows now. She works on how angry she is at herself for her earlier drinking and then feels self-compassion as she recognizes what led her to drink. In the process of this exploration, she increases her ability to put her complex feelings about this issue into words. She also recognizes that it will take courage to bring up the topic with her son again and that she will be risking rejection because he is angry. Eventually, she initiates a conversation in which she tells him about her former problems drinking, her regrets about it, and the strength it took to stop. She reminds him of his many strengths and conveys her belief that he, too, can stop. She comes into therapy reporting that she does not know what the upshot of this conversation will be, but she knows it was important to have it. She grows tearful. We both know the work she did to have that conversation. She faced shame and regret, the painful recognition that there is no redoing, the embarrassment of exposure and the risk that her son would reject her. This was a meaningful expression of her love.

I am aware as I write this that I, too, seek meaning. I am deeply moved when I see my patients use their therapy to engage with life in ways that provide meaning. Their doing so provides *me* with a sense my life has meaning. I am grateful to have the opportunity to do this work.

Letting go, "relinquishing" omnipotence, and surrender with agency

I have put the word relinquishing in quotes because, with Searles (1965), I do not believe one "resolves" omnipotence. Each of us harbors a self-state in which we continue to experience ourselves as omnipotent. We enter a state of disbelief when this self is confronted with mortality, when we feel our powerlessness. We are shocked, outraged, and despair when our omnipotence fails. "Never, never, never, never, never." King Lear cries out these words, holding his daughter's dead body, in one of the most devastating scenes in theater. Lear speaks for all of us. The dead will not return to life. Never. And, like Lear, we cry out in anguish and anger when we face that. I believe the popularity of Dylan Thomas' famous line, "Rage, rage against the dying of the light" results from his speaking for this universal part of human experience.

Humankind, *homo faber*, has been long defined by our species' tool use (although recent naturalistic observation has robbed us of this unique distinction!) We are the animals who transcend the limits of environment by inventing the wheel, the engine, and the antibiotic. If the human striving is for control, however, we must also face our lack of it. We may fly planes and erect skyscrapers, but we cannot get our 2-year-olds to go to bed. And we die. King Lear cannot bring Cordelia back to life. Humans are not omnipotent but a part of our being believes we should be.

We do better when we do not silence this part of ourselves. Rather our best bet is to feel and acknowledge our powerful needs for magical control, our steadfast belief that we can control, and then to broker an entente between those parts of ourselves and the more reality-related portions of our beings. Brokering this entente is an active process, requiring psychological work. Throughout a life there are often periods where one achieves an equilibrium, managing to feel empowered while recognizing one's lack of control. Then life presents challenges that jeopardize this equilibrium. Facing one's mortality in older age is one of these occasions. No matter that you have reached a degree of emotional maturity in which you have accepted your lack of omnipotence – facing death will put that to the test. One must then reckon with the cruelest of narcissistic blows: one will die.

Mitchell (1986), building on Nietzsche's concept of "tragic man," describes two undesirable solutions to the problem of living within the limits imposed by reality: One can live as if there are no limits or one can be deadened by these limits. He illustrates these solutions with the image of a man on the beach with the tide coming in. If he constructs elaborate sandcastles believing they will last forever, he will be devastated when they are destroyed by the tide. If, on the other hand, he is so depleted by recognizing the reality of the tide that he refrains from creating anything, he ends up with an empty beach. Nietzsche's tragic man, Mitchell explains, takes neither of these routes. He is aware of the tide yet builds anyway. "The inevitable limitations of reality do not dim the passion in which he builds his castles; in fact, the inexorable realities add a poignancy and sweetness to his passion" (p. 120). This is the solution that Freud (1916) recommended in his essay on transience. This is Shakespeare's "to love that well which thou must leave ere long." This is the solution that we would hope for older adults: To face death realistically, yet to remain creatively invested in life. Yet this resolution is hard to maintain in older age, since the experience of helplessness in the face of mortality can be crushing.

How does the animal who invented the lever, the light bulb, and the nuclear bomb accept that there is absolutely nothing he can do about dying? Ultimately one must face the inevitable and surrender. Surrender,

Ghent (1990) wrote, need not entail humiliating defeat. Rather it can be an expression of letting go and of expansion of the self, bringing "a sense of wholeness, even one's sense of unity with other living beings" (p. 111). Bach (2019) elaborates on this idea, positing that there are two types of surrender. In the pathological form, one is overwhelmed, surrendering personal agency. In the creative form, in contrast, one remains an actor by an active process, including self-observation, self-experiencing, and self-refueling. Surrender in this view requires relinquishing omnipotence but not agency. The older adult who is actively engaged in understanding the experience of her final years, who is still working on her relationships, and who is finding ways to give to others – even if all she can give is her great gratitude for their care – retains her agency even as her control over her body diminishes, even as she faces death.

As Beethoven composed his last quartet, he penned in German above one musical theme, "Must it be?" and above a second, "It must be!" Some lovers of Beethoven, recognizing the sublime, spiritual depth of his quartets, believe that he was facing death with his question and accepting it with his response. (Other theories abound, including that he was repeating the words of a recent monetary transaction!) If these words were indeed an expression of feelings about mortality, Beethoven's response might be seen as the creative surrender Ghent and Bach describe. For while in the very act of facing and accepting death, he was actively immersed in creating a quartet. Let us not forget, however, that in writing his quartet, in the act of surrendering, Beethoven was still voicing a protest: "Must it be?" Surrender is neither a passive act nor a one-time affair. Rather, it is an active process that must be achieved, only with effort, repeatedly.

How do psychotherapists help their patients with this task of surrendering to the inevitable while retaining the sense of self as agent? Much of the work of therapy described earlier addresses this issue obliquely. Increasing one's understanding of oneself and of others, finding ways to participate in life which provide a sense of meaning, experiencing one's resilience in finding new answers to old problems – all these enhance one' experience of agency as one faces life's end. At times, however, the issue comes up more directly and dramatically as wishes for an omnipotent rescuer enter the therapeutic relationship.

The older patient is slammed with harsh realities about the end of life. Omnipotent longings, even if long subdued, may be aroused and brought to the therapist in the form of a wish that the therapist bestow omnipotence.

A hidden agenda emerges: "Therapist, stop this suffering. Make me immortal." When a patient can feel these wishes and the immense disappointment and anger that comes with the therapist's failure to provide, and when a therapist can meet these feelings authentically, the two are joined in a potent moment of vital connection. Patient and therapist together recognize their human helpless in the face of death, mourn what the therapist cannot provide and are united in their experience of surrender with agency. These are examples of Buber's "I-Thou" relatedness (Buber, 1970), and they can be thought of as the "moments of meeting" that researchers now identify as catalysts of change (Boston Change Study Group, 1998). I lived through just such a powerful moment with Jean

Jean

Soon to turn 80, Jean was a capable woman who prided herself on her efficiency and competence. Although she complained about her husband's and adult children's dependence on her, she was insightful enough to recognize that she also liked it that way and that she had set up their lives so she could feel in charge. Then life started handing her situations she couldn't handle. Here's one of many. Her husband, suffering a degenerative neurological disease and newly disabled, fell out of bed and could not get up. She discovered that she wasn't strong enough to help him up. Nobody she knew was close enough to call and it made no sense to call 911, she told me, just because someone had fallen out of bed. Eventually she went out into the street and prevailed upon a new neighbor for help. She was quite resourceful in doing that and her engaging personality plus good social skills allowed her not only to get help but to make it a pleasant encounter. Meanwhile, her husband could no longer do many of the tasks he had performed in the past. Using the defenses she had relied on since childhood, instead of feeling the losses and the dependency needs which were revived in this situation, Jean dissociated these feelings and moved into a super-efficient, caretaking mode. This, however, left her angry and angry at herself for feeling angry. She then suffered a major depressive episode, losing weight because she had no appetite, deeply despairing. Medication did not help. This was the background that led to the following session.

"I have a check for you," stated Jean, "but I don't feel like giving it to you. I'm angry." She then added, "I'm not planning to leave, but I need to ask this." There followed a long pause as she leaned forward and looked directly into my eyes. Then she uttered, with pauses between each sentence and with the vocal intensity of a howl: "Why am I here? You can't restore my husband's body or mind. You can't keep him from dying. You can't keep me from dying. And you can't help me walk without pain. You can't make my life better. Why am I here?" Although her words in themselves were questions, her tone of voice and body posture made them a protest, a powerful one, about my inability to keep her and her husband safe. The total silence that followed required a response. I knew that an interpretation would be distancing, was not what was needed. And I felt pierced by the knowledge that what Jean most wanted from me I could not give. I had little time for thought. Spontaneously, and with an emotional intensity matching hers, I answered, "I don't want you to go through this alone." The answer came from my heart and she knew it. We sat silently, taking it all in.

Jean's communication had more than one meaning. On one level, our work was about repetition and can be seen as a transference communication. On this level, we can look at Jean as having accessed a previously dissociated affective state, as having accessed a well of feelings about her unmet needs in childhood. These were no longer split off, could be integrated into her felt self and expressed in the here-and-now of our relationship. She fervently desired me to ameliorate the painful and frightening conditions in her life; she was angry and disappointed that I was not helping. That she was able to tell me this and that she could do so with such feeling was important. She had been the good, non-complaining child of over-burdened parents. She, who had had a "difficult" older sibling, had been the child who had tried to need nothing. Now she was allowing herself to feel her wishes and to register pain and anger at their being unmet. She, who had been a lifelong caretaker to others, seeking little for herself, was newly able to feel her own desires and deprivations and to speak them out loud.

My response in the moment did not address the transferential aspect of Jean's communication. Instinctively I felt that meeting her on another level felt more important. My choice here brings to mind S. Stern's (2017) distinction between needed relationships and repeated relationships and his concern that relational psychoanalysis has over-emphasized the latter. Yes, Jean's comment can be seen as addressing a repeated relationship: Once again she had a parental figure who was failing her. But more important, I sensed, was her request for a needed relationship in the present. Jean had uttered a howl of existential anguish. "How can it be that I will die, and that you cannot help?" She was reckoning with her mortality. My spontaneous response met this existential cry in the only way we can. I could not rebut her recognition of how little I could do for her in the face of disability and death. Instead, in Levenkron's (2009) words, "I did what I felt to be the human thing" (p. 187). I offered all that we can offer (not nothing). We were two mortals, facing this together.

In the weeks that followed we talked about what therapy could and could not offer and together mourned what it could not. We talked about death, her lack of belief in an afterlife. We talked about uncertainty. Neither of us knew how long we would live. Neither of us knew when or how the end would come. I said to Jean, "For us to work together, both of us have to live with the painful feelings of how much I cannot do for you." I also said to her, "It's true, I can't protect you from dying. I can't protect myself from dying either." We both registered the truth and the sadness of this state of affairs.

We also talked about her childhood. Jean has almost no recollection of childhood events. Mostly she remembers feeling states: loneliness, invisibility, recognizing that there was nobody around to help and fear, always fear. Jean's parents had suffered significant trauma before their immigration from Eastern Europe. Like many of their generation described by Hahn (2019), they never spoke of what they had endured. Instead there was silence. The unmetabolized ordeals contributed significantly to the affects predominant in Jean's home, resulting in intergenerational transmission of trauma. There were few words for feelings back then; that was the realm of unmentalized affectivity, of emotions that had never been identified or put into words (Jurist, 2018). But now Jean began to experience similar emotions of fear, anger, helplessness, and need. And this time, she could feel them and speak them.

As we did this work, Jean reported a startling change in herself. Her major depressive episode vanished and suddenly, at the age of 79, she found herself shedding her long-standing self-denying, caretaking approach to life. She obtained sufficient help in the home that her husband could receive the care he needed without her sacrificing herself. She marveled at a newly felt freedom to spend money on herself and to treat herself to a lunch out. No longer constricting her emotional life, she found herself more open with friends and more expressive of affection to her grandchildren. She surprised herself with her ability to savor the good parts of her life, even as she lived with the painful parts and knew that more difficult times were to come. "I can't believe it," she said, "I'm feeling joy."

Jean had been in psychoanalysis earlier in her life and, while benefitting from it, had also learned how incremental change can be. Now, lifelong patterns were shifting rapidly. "What's happening that I'm changing so quickly?" Jean asked.

I don't have an answer to Jean's question. I speculate, however, that something about the synchrony of existential and early-childhood issues in older patients magnifies the power of our work. For many people, the rigors of later life may awaken long-dormant states of being. Dissociated experience can finally be refelt, expressed and integrated in a painful but revitalizing process. Bromberg (1998) tells us, "it is humanly impossible to become fully alive in the present without facing and owning all the hated, disavowed parts of the self . . ." (p. 6). Feeling the feelings of long-dissociated affect-laden experience allowed Jean to become fully alive. Meanwhile, since older adults often have a combination of strengths, resilience and insight born of life experience which together permit for highly effective work on that which has reemerged, this work brought significant rewards. That is why a little goes a long way in our work with older adults. Even in a short time, people can grow enormously.

References

Alpert, J. L. (2012). Loss of humanness: The ultimate trauma. *The American Journal of Psychoanalysis, 72*(2), 118–138.

American Psychiatric Association. (2013). *Diagnostic and statistical manual of mental disorders* (5th ed.). American Psychiatric Association.

Bach, S. (2019). States of self-surrender. *Psychoanalytic Psychology, 36*(2), 159–165.

Becker, E. (1973). *The denial of death*. The Free Press.

Boston Change Study Group. (1998). Non-interpretive mechanisms in psychoanalytic therapy. *International Journal of Psycho-Analysis, 79*, 903–921.

Brody, S. (2016). *Entering night country: Psychoanalytic reflections on loss and resilience*. Routledge.

Bromberg, P. M. (1998). *Standing in the spaces*. Analytic Press.

Buber, M. (1970). *I and thou*. Scribner.

Clement, C. (2005). The evocation of death anxiety on a meditation retreat. *Psychoanalytic Dialogues, 15*(2), 139–152.

Cooper, S. H. (2016). *The analyst's experience of the depressive position: The melancholic errand of psychoanalysis*. Routledge.

Freud, S. (1916). On transience. In J. Strachey (Ed. & Trans.), *The standard edition of the complete psychological works of Sigmund Freud* (Vol. 14, pp. 303–307). Hogarth Press.

Frommer, M. (2005). Concepts of self and the impact of loss: Reply to commentaries. *Psychoanalytic Dialogues, 15*(4), 549–557.

Ghent, E. (1990). Masochism, submission, surrender – Masochism as a perversion of surrender. *Contemporary Psychoanalysis, 26,* 108–136.

Hahn, H. (2019). *They left it all behind: Trauma, loss and memory among Eastern European Jewish immigrants and their children.* Rowman & Littlefield.

Jurist, E. (2018). *Minding emotions: Cultivating mentalization in psychotherapy.* Guilford Press.

Lev, G. (2016). The question of aims: Psychoanalysis and the changing formulations of the life worth living. *Psychoanalytic Psychology, 33*(2), 312–333.

Levenkron, H. (2009). Engaging the implicit: Meeting points between the Boston change process study group and relational psychoanalysis. *Contemporary Psychoanalysis, 45*(2), 179–217.

Lifton, R. J. (1979). *The broken connection.* Simon & Schuster.

Mitchell, S. A. (1986). The wings of Icarus: Illusion and the problem of narcissism. *Contemporary Psychoanalysis, 22,* 107–132.

Searles, H. F. (1965). *Collected papers on schizophrenia and other subjects.* International Universities Press.

Slavin, M. O. (2016). Relational psychoanalysis and the tragic-existential aspect of the human condition. *Psychoanalytic Dialogues, 26*(5), 537–548.

Solomon, S., Greenberg, J., & Pyszczynski, T. (2015). *The worm at the core: On the role of death in life.* Penguin Books.

Stern, S. (2017). *Needed relationships and psychoanalytic healing: A holistic relational perspective on the therapeutic process.* Routledge.

Symington, N. (2006). *A healing conversation: How healing happens.* Karnac.

Yalom, I. D. (1980). *Existential psychotherapy.* Basic Books.

Yalom, I. D. (2008). *Staring at the sun: Overcoming the terror of death.* Jossey-Bass.

Chapter 7

Endings

Anna:	"I'm making a list of who to notify when I die and their phone numbers." She quickly moves on to another topic. I wait for a pause and then ask:
Amy:	"Am I on the list?"
Anna:	"Yes." She pauses. "Thank you for asking."
Amy:	"I would want to know."
Anna:	"Thank you." Another longer pause.
Amy:	"I hope it won't be for a long time from now, that things go well for you and that you enjoy your life before then . . . but I want you to know that I will miss you very much when that happens."
Anna, in tears:	"Thank you. Thank you for telling me."
Amy:	I nod. I am in tears, too.

Anna, in her late 80s, was still functioning fully, but she had several serious physical conditions. In a recent medical visit, she spoke frankly to a physician she trusted. "As one professional to another," she said, "how much time would you give me?" The doctor answered. "You could go on for another 2–3 years. But given what's happening with your (name of organs), you could also pop off at any time." Anna had already guessed that. Our conversation took place shortly after that. And I was filled with grief.

This chapter is about endings: the endings of lives, the endings of treatments, and the end of this book. I will start, however, with openings, changes precipitated by endings which contribute to growth toward the end of life. I will move to mourning, looking first at our patients' mourning, then at our own. I will close with Anna, with whom the earlier conversation took place. My work with her is now permeated with the realities, affects, and complications of endings.

One type of ending I will omit because (fortunately) I have not experienced it. It is the loss of a patient to suicide. The topic of suicide among patients of all ages is sadly under-addressed in our literature (Tillman & Carter, 2014). It is a particularly important topic in the treatment of elders because of their high suicide rate. And it is a complex topic because geriatricians report an increasing number of older adults who manifest no signs of mental illness and who are not terminally ill but wish to take matters into their own hands and end their lives, while they are still doing well (Balasubramaniam, 2018). Baby Boomers, they say, are used to controlling their lives and wish to control their deaths as well. The psychological, social, philosophical, and ethical aspects of this trend will be of interest to those treating older adults.

Openings at an ending

"Openings at an ending" is the expression that Gerson (2018) uses to describes the psychological changes consequent to the death of one's parent. She proposes that while psychoanalytic writings tend to portray internal parental representations as stable, these representations are in fact fluid and can be altered by the powerful experiences accompanying the death of a parent. A similar phenomenon can occur in later life. The potent experiences of facing their own deaths can propel older adults into comparable "openings at an ending." The corresponding transformations of their internal worlds can be striking.

"There has to be a statute of limitations on how one's mother and father failed as people or parents," states Burack-Weiss (2015, p. 87), describing the way she and a number of noted authors have, in older age, changed their perceptions of their parents. The same phenomenon, the improved relationships with the people inhabiting one's inner world, is reported by Quindoz (2010), who identifies this alteration as part of the reparative process of the depressive position. Repeatedly, I have found my older patients modifying their views of long-dead parents. Even those who have had previous psychodynamic therapy, and therefore have already examined their early relationships in some depth, manifest these changes. Often the change consists of a lessening of condemnation, as described by Burack-Weiss and Quindoz. Sometimes, in contrast, the modification of perception entails a new recognition of flaws. In almost all cases, it is the transformation of a simpler picture into one more complex, often one imbued with compassion. This transformation may evoke strong feelings, as insight and memory combine to bring recognition of the pain borne both by the self and by the parent in episodes of childhood difficulty.

What accounts for this shift? Hoffman (1998) reports the results of his study of parents who have lost a child to leukemia. He was impressed by how many of them matured, exhibiting "a greater empathic identification with and tolerance for the limitations of others and an enhanced sense of resiliency and capacity to endure suffering" (p. 62). He concludes that facing mortality can evoke growth. Older adults face their mortality and as they experience their own increased frailty, they may acquire greater compassion for the frailties of others. Fearsome parents are no longer seen as all-powerful but rather as fallible mortals. In addition, older adults' longer-range perspectives and the process of elaborating their own life stories afford the appreciation of greater complexity, allowing more complex views of multifaceted parents. Having to face and metabolize their own regrets, too, may help them tolerate the imperfections of others. Therapy fosters mentalization, the capacity to understand the minds of self and others. This capacity, too, may lead to a greater understanding of the complex motivations which led to a parents' injurious behavior, perhaps changing the impact of the injury. Hunter (1999) quotes an 82-year-old patient describing this experience: "I feel now differently toward my mother. I can see how unhappy she was – she must have been desperately unhappy – my attitude toward her has mellowed. When my time comes I don't think I'll take so much bitterness with me" (p. 242).

The sequelae of these alterations of the patient's object representations, of the cast of characters which make up their inner worlds, are important. Greater acceptance of the parent is often accompanied by greater acceptance of the self, weakening an old object tie which might be called, "bad mother-bad self." These changes reduce the use of the primitive defense of splitting, the defense in which good and bad are sharply delineated, permitting no synthesis. Horwitz (2005), in a plea for psychoanalysts to engage more with the concept of forgiveness, describes this process. One can let go of intense negative feelings toward the parent, he says, by seeing their offences in the context of the whole person, perhaps even developing empathy for what motivated the parent's hurtful behavior. Instead of splitting, one can see the parent as an integrated person. The end result may also be something we have trouble defining and seldom talk about: wisdom.

Although elders are often seen as isolated, vivid memories of others may offer at least some of what was formerly provided by actual living people. Galatzer-Levy and Cohler (1990) describe these memories as playing self-object functions that "support a person's sense of liveliness and cohesiveness" (p. 94). Older adults' more nuanced and resonant perceptions of others long gone may, therefore, bestow a more sustaining and nourishing internal environment that meets social-emotional needs even when an individual is alone. This transformation of the inner world may also be helpful in facing one's finitude. As Bergmann (2014) notes, "It is our capacity to have good internal objects that enables us to accept death" (p. 241). Openings at the ending, the alteration of internal representations, may therefore have multiple beneficial effects.

Mourning

There has been a revision in the psychoanalytic understanding of mourning, a change of such magnitude that Hagman (2016) calls current theory "new mourning." Among the contributors to the development of this new view are analysts whose own experiences of mourning led them to recognize the limitations of extant theory and to expand on it. Hagman, whose wrenching story of his father's death identifies him as a member of that group, provides a description and critique of the earlier model of mourning. Then, pulling together the work of others and adding his own conclusions, he offers the following more contemporary view. Each mourning process is unique – there is no "standard" sequence of stages. Harm can be done by a misguided adherence to a prescribed model, for example when mourners are pushed into expressing grief by well-meaning professionals. Mourning is a social, intersubjective, process and cannot be done in isolation. The survivor needs others for holding, for help bearing overwhelming affect, for meeting narcissistic needs, for feeling connection, and for putting complex experiences into words. The goal is not, as formerly thought, the de-cathecting of, but rather the transformation of, the internal relationship with the lost object. The process is one aimed toward restoring the continuity of self-experience by reorganizing the survivor's sense of self and self-in-relation. Its aim is to preserve meaning.

The patient mourns

Losses multiply in older age. Older adults bear a lifetime of past and current losses as they face the largest loss of all – the endings of their own lives. Current losses, moreover, revitalize the pain of earlier losses. Mourning thus becomes a major task in one's later years. It requires effort. In Buechler's (2019) words, "Bearing loss can take all we have, every ounce of strength, every source of inspiration and determination" (p. 47). Yet this work and the need for it may be dismissed by others. Older adults may be surrounded by people who believe they are helping by encouraging their elders to get past a loss quickly. Peskin (2019), discussing the social ranking of states of grief, comments, "Mourning for the elderly, including elders mourning the death of each other, occupies a lower ranking of grief in popular culture. . . . Between their accumulated grief of a lifetime and holding back their grief for their families' sake, elder mourners both create and join the perception that late loss has small value" (p. 488). A colleague in her 80s tells me that a mere few months after her husband's death friends, including fellow psychotherapists, were telling her it was time to "move on." Sometimes the therapist's office is the only place where elders' grief is taken seriously.

Many aspects of psychodynamic psychotherapy discussed in earlier chapters aid the mourning process. The empathic, witnessing psychotherapist helps the patient bear the unbearable affects of intense grief. Feelings are put into words – and since some of these feelings may be socially unacceptable or be accompanied by shame, talking with the psychotherapist may provide an opportunity for full self-expression impossible with other mourners. The "ghosts" of early abandonments revived can be recognized as coming from the past and mourned or re-mourned along with the current loss. In addition, feelings accompanying the experience of loss, such as regret, which may complicate or hinder the mourning process, can be worked with. "Why were my last words to him not more loving, why was I impatient?" a patient might say. This regret and the pain over the human lack of omniscience – she did not know these would be the last words – must be recognized and lived with.

One does not "resolve" grief. Freud (1929), in contradiction to his theoretical writing on mourning, knew that. In a letter, he wrote on the anniversary of his daughter's death to Ludwig Binswanger, who had just lost a son, he said, "We know that the acute sorrow we feel after such a loss will run its course, but also that we will remain inconsolable, and will never find a substitute" (p. 196).

The pain of loss may abate with time, but one does not "get over" loss, for it may permanently change the self. Careful evidence of this change is provided by Notman (2014), who observed and then wrote about her own widowhood. One's self-concept changes along with one's social status. One's future self, an envisioned "going on being" connected to the other, is irredeemably altered. And the parts of the self that were shared only with the other, known only to the other, are gone.

The therapist who understands this, who has patience with the process, and who does not expect the patient to "get back to normal," slowly fosters the development of a reorganized sense of self. Gradually the self-narrative gets rewritten, knitting together the old with the incomprehensible new reality and the newly envisioned future. Often patients see their former history in a new light as they look back on it from the vantage point of current loss. Their life story must then be retold. Putting this story into words, having these words heard and held by the therapist, helps the patient develop a new and more complex self-narrative one which strengthens self-continuity in the face of loss. The self may be bereft forever, but it goes on. Patients may eventually be able to say, "I am hurting and sad and I'll never be the same, but I'm still me." Perhaps this is what Quindoz (2010) means when she talks about "Losing everything without losing oneself" (p. 77).

The death of a loved one may precipitate not only loss but also an onslaught of existential anguish and a desolate sense of meaninglessness. The reminder of mortality brings into sharp relief the absurdity of life. We are born. We spend some time on the planet thinking that what we do has some importance. Then we die and are gone. What in the world was it all about? These issues arise for any mourner, but particularly so in older adults who must reckon with loss in the context of facing their own life's extinction. One of the tasks of the late-life mourner is to reestablish a sense of life's meaning. In Chapter 6, I discussed routes to the experience of meaning in later life. In the process of mourning, this experience is also fostered by recognizing one's own desolation as part of the human condition and by feeling a kinship with other fellow sufferers. The work in therapy to feel rather than dissociate and to deepen intimacy in relationships fosters this process. The heightening of compassion for self and others that accompanies growth in therapy does this as well.

The therapist mourns

Immersed in the intense experience of facing mortality, older patients and their therapists often forge deep, intimate bonds. When a bond of this depth is ruptured, how does the therapist mourn?

Buechler (2012) discusses the impact on therapists of their successive terminations, their chronic mourning. She believes these unending losses have much more impact than is recognized. She even speculates that the warfare between psychoanalytic schools could be due to aggression provoked by the unprocessed grief of analysts. Chronic mourning is, no doubt, an issue for all therapists. It is, however, a particularly difficult challenge for the therapists of older adults. For us, the losses come not merely from termination but too often from disability or death. In addition, some of our grief stems not only from actual deaths but also from those anticipated. The snippet of a session with which I started this chapter left me with intense feelings about the loss that had not yet happened.

Terminations

Terminations of older adults may affect us in unique ways. True, we mourn the end of treatment no matter the age of the patient. When we terminate with younger patients, however, we may carry sustaining fantasies of what their futures may hold. The connection with their imagined future keeps the tie alive and may even soothe. As Silverman (2010) notes, "Loss, when held meaningfully, when held in the context of an inner sense of going-on-being, has a way of providing not only pain but comfort" (p. 188). With older patients going on being is in question. A fantasized future does not sustain the tie and the loss is that much keener.

A mutually planned termination, therapists would agree, is optimal. Both parties recognize it is a good time to stop, they review their work together, they value their accomplishments, they express and examine multiple levels of feelings from present and past, and they say goodbye. Such terminations can constitute a poignant and nourishing processes for both therapist and patient. If only this type of termination were always possible! With older adults there are so many other – much less satisfying – endings.

A patient's death

"Like sexuality, grief can be requited or unrequited – for sexuality by being loved, for grief by being solaced" writes Peskin (2019, p. 478). Most often the therapist's grief upon a patient's death is unrequited. The therapist, like every human being who loses an intimate relationship, must mourn. But how? Even if he can attend the patient's funeral, the therapist, the "undesignated mourner" (Aronson, 2009), mourns alone. Yet mourning alone is an oxymoron. Mourning requires a social environment of co-mourners and social rituals play psychological functions fostering mourning (Slochower, 1993). In most cases, the bereaved therapist has access to neither. The therapist therefore faces a double tragedy: a death and the absence of a way to mourn.

Literature by analysts whose patients have died is often poignant and powerful, describing how isolating and distressing the experience can be. Richards (2013), after learning that a boy she had previously treated had been murdered, says, "The knowledge haunted me and eventually led me to give up my child therapy practice altogether" (p. 93). She adds, "I could not bear my grief because I could not really share it" (p. 93). Adelman (2013) writes that after a patient's sudden death, "I was alone, silenced and silently devastated by the loss of my patient" (p. 84).

A patient's death may also evoke complicated feelings, such as shame or guilt, which increase the challenge of mourning. Therapists may experience shame when they worry about loss of income, judging themselves inhumane to be thinking about money when someone has died. Survivor's guilt may torment, too: What right do I have to be alive when my patient is not? Therapists may worry that the extent of their grief is unprofessional. Daehnert (2008), for example, attributed a period of immobilization after treating a dying patient to the shame she felt over how deeply moved she was by the treatment. What is more, the omnipotent fantasies therapists often bring to their work with elders – which, Frommer (2016) suggests, sustain them in their efforts – can lead to feelings of failure. The therapist of the deceased patient has failed to keep the patient alive. Marshall (2008), whose patient died in a car accident, suffered because she had not protected her patient from what was coming. Magical thinking, she tells us, led her to feel overtaken by guilt. How heavy such feelings make the burden of the therapist's mourning!

Ambiguous losses and living with uncertainty

Ambiguous loss (Boss, 2000) is the loss that evades closure. This is the kind of loss adult children suffer as they watch a parent's advancing dementia. The person is both gone and not gone. How do you say goodbye to someone who is still there? A debilitating stroke that abolishes speech or a coma can end the treatment of an older adult suddenly and with no opportunity for termination. In these cases, therapy is clearly no longer possible although the patient still lives. This is one kind of unhappy ending, an ending that defies the comfort of closure.

Therapists, however, are often up against a second type of unhappy ending, one even more difficult to mourn. There are a host of situations in which it is not clear whether it is necessary to end. A patient's problems with cognition, hearing, mobility, sedating medications, and pain – any of these may interfere enough with the therapy process that questions arise. Can we keep going? Do we need a break or is this the end? Is psychotherapy still useful or am I deluding myself to avoid letting go? What is in the patient's best interest? And how can the therapist's needs be considered? Buechler (2019) discusses the degree of shame therapists may feel when their self-interest is involved. Therapists forced to decide whether their already taxing schedules can now encompass regular home visits to homebound patients, forced to face the conflict between their patients' needs and their own, may feel that shame. Caregivers' needs and preferences may also enter the equation and sometimes it is the caregiver rather than therapist or patient who ends up making the decision. Despite our best intentions, our endings with older adults may be far from ideal and haunted by uncertainty.

"For all flesh is as grass . . . and the flower thereof falleth away." These are the words, accompanied by exquisitely haunting music, of Brahms Requiem. Work with older adults brings with it the aches that attend endings, the repeated losses of those we may have grown to love. And it teaches that lives (and treatments) end in messy, unpredictable, ways. Yet even as we mourn these losses, we can be sustained by the fulfillment of having witnessed our patients' late-life growth. December flowers may fall away, but what a joy that they bloomed.

Reflections on ending: Anna

As I approach the ending of this book, I find myself looking back over its various chapters and reviewing the therapeutic journey undertaken by older patients. I will now briefly revisit ideas I have presented earlier. To illustrate these, I will turn to Anna, with whom I started this chapter – Anna who was making a list of the people to inform when she dies. Telling the story of her treatment allows me both to savor the fruitfulness of our work together and to illustrate the way these ideas apply to her progress in therapy. It will also help with my grief as I face the possible/probable end of our work together.

How to describe Anna? I can start with her severe early trauma. Premature, she spent her early month first in an incubator, then in a hospital – this in the days when parental visits were not allowed. Her family life was chaotic with a violent father who disappeared periodically, a mother who resourcefully held the family together by holding two jobs, and her own parentified role as she did the housework and cared for several younger siblings at an early age. Periodically, when her mother was overwhelmed, she was sent away to stay with relatives she hardly knew. I can also talk of Anna's impressive resilience. With this background, with parents who had never finished high school, she eventually obtained a graduate degree and a responsible job in market research. She married an accountant, had three children, assumed an upper middle-class lifestyle – and was utterly miserable.

Anna first came to me in her 50s, 30 years ago. With children grown, she was depressed and considering leaving her husband. She made good use of her therapy. Her marital situation improved considerably, her life was much better and after 9 years she terminated with an understanding that she could come back as needed. For the next decade, she stayed in touch, coming in every year or two for a few sessions. She was doing fine.

Then, as she approached 80, it all fell apart. Life handed her misfortunes. She was beset by several physical ailments that were intermittently painful, required surgery and medical monitoring, and had the potential to kill. Her husband, with beginning dementia and following a stroke, needed care and suffered severe mood swings. She felt isolated as siblings and friends either died or moved away. This formerly resilient, confident professional had been transformed into a tiny, physically frail, self-hating, isolated woman in great distress. We began weekly phone sessions.

In Chapter 2, "Ghosts in Later Life," I focused on how older adults reencounter earlier developmental challenges and the way these revive earlier relational conflicts. In Anna's case, the need to rework her solutions to earlier developmental challenges was heralded by the multiple painful bruises she had acquired tumbling down her steep cellar steps with a loaded laundry basket. "I thought I had broken something," she told me, "but luckily I'm just badly bruised. I'll have to be more careful when I do the laundry next week." I listened in horror, visualizing this frail, medically compromised woman lugging laundry up and down steep stairs. While not without financial concerns, Anna could have easily paid for someone to do her laundry. I asked why she was risking life and limb to do it herself.

Anna's fall had shaken her up enough that she was open to exploring what was behind her desire to handle everything alone. An issue we had touched on before, her need to experience herself as self-reliant, now acquired new urgency. Anna began to look anew at earlier developmental challenges surrounding trust and autonomy. Her childhood had left her with little basic trust and a brittle autonomy which would allow for no vulnerability. One of her earliest memories is of figuring out a way to wash out her panties unobserved after an "accident," this before she was in kindergarten. Striving for self-sufficiency had given her an illusion of safety in an unreliable world and a feeling of control rather than powerlessness. It had also allowed her to disavow emotions that would have threatened her attachment to her mother, such as her powerful yearnings to be taken care of and rage over deprivations and abandonments. With her dependency needs disowned, her capacity to go it alone had served her well under difficult circumstances. But now the defenses marshalled to keep at bay the powerful feelings evoked by her need for help were endangering her life. For her own safety, she needed to find new solutions to old issues.

In Chapter 3, "Trauma and Trauma Redux," I discussed the way late-life trauma can reawaken the affects of earlier traumatic episodes. Anna's current physical pain, frailty, need to depend on others, exposure to her husband's periodic temper outbursts, and her multiple losses all served to revive trauma from earlier eras of her life. She reexperienced long-dissociated self-states involving powerful feelings of helplessness, terror, rage, shame, and self-loathing. These could now be shared, put into words, and understood. Anna realized, for example, that her husband was physically incapable of harming her and that the panic she felt when he raised his voice sprang from traumatic early episodes when her father's violent rages had terrorized the family.

Anna was now immersed in distressing affects that stemmed both from her current life and from early trauma. Our work on this twofold experience led to significant change. For Anna became able to feel long-dissociated desires for nurturance. Eventually she was able to cry to me, "I've taken care of so many people all my life; why is nobody taking care of me?"

In Chapter 4, "*Dramatis Personae*, Past and Present," I examined how early family relationships are relived with the therapist. In the transference, I joined the cast of characters from Anna's early trauma. Sometimes, I was the rescuer she had always longed for. But then that would switch. In a last session before my vacation, for example, she said with a mock seriousness which did not disguise the underlying feeling, "You know that you're not allowed to leave, don't you?" I was now her abandoning mother. In our earlier years of working together, Anna had never felt or expressed such feelings. Now, as she was able to feel what she had long dissociated, she began to relax her crusade for self-sufficiency and to tolerate the dependency on others required by her disabilities. She found people to help with household chores and the care of her husband, engaging them for trial periods so that she could select the reliable ones. She then established comfortable relationships with these helpers and enjoyed their company. As I explained in Chapter 2, Anna's contact with long-buried feelings from her past, while temporarily destabilizing, did not constitute a regression. Rather, Anna was able to integrate these feelings and then to exercise a more flexible autonomy which permitted her to seek help. Her capable, adult functioning allowed her to do this effectively. And she no longer carried heavy loads of laundry up and down the stairs.

In Chapter 5, "The Narration of Life Stories and the Self," I wrote about the ways therapy helps to transform the life narrative and strengthen the self. Together, Anna and I were rewriting Anna's story. Weaving together present and past, we were creating a new narrative. Her old story line was one of triumph over hardship via self-reliance and a precipitous late-life plunge into debased dependence. Her new, more complex, story line recognized her adaptiveness. Striving for self-sufficiency had been adaptive in early life and took her far. Flexibly relinquishing this stance as she needed assistance was adaptive now and allowed for more comfort in her later years. Anna experienced agency as she took delight in this new perspective. Her fuller self-narrative helped to strengthen Anna's sense of self and counter the narcissistic damage wrought by so much loss – of her career, her siblings, the physical strength, and the independence which had been sources of pride. Anna now found her inner life interesting and appreciated the strengths through which she overcame difficulties. She began to like herself again and to look back on her life as valuable.

There was one sticking point, however, one facet of Anna's life which still soured her self-regard. In Chapter 5, we saw that moral injury, the harm one has done to others, can undermine a positive life narrative. Anna was deeply troubled by the way she had been treating her physically and cognitively disabled husband. His periods of lucidity were punctuated by angry episodes in which he demanded services of her which were impossible. Anna could not stop herself from screaming insults at him. Yet she hated herself every time she did it. "What kind of person is mean to someone who is brain-damaged and can't help himself?" she asked. Eventually, she realized that she screamed at her husband because she believed him. Memories returned of the times when her exhausted mother gave her responsibilities that were far beyond her young capabilities. To better deal with her husband, she needed to quiet a battle between the internalized mother's voice telling she could do it all and the part of herself still angry at being asked to do the impossible. Gradually, she was able to stop screaming. She adopted a method of saying quietly as she left his room, "I'll be back when you're calmer." And she also began to exhibit greater self-compassion, recognizing that an occasional sharp word in response to her husband's behavior was only human.

In Chapter 6, "Existential Anxieties," I examined three existential tasks faced by older adults: the search for meaning, facing one's lack of omnipotence, and the transition to death as a felt experience. Anna worked on all these issues. As she grew less reactive to her husband's anger, she began to reflect more, wondering aloud in a session if her husband's belligerence came from feeling emasculated. His vision was failing; he needed a cane and had become incontinent. In our next session, she told me that instead of leaving the room when he had shouted, she had sat next to him and said, "I think we're both having a very hard time with old age." He grew calmer and told her that he felt he had been abandoned by God. Holding hands, they then talked quietly about aging and death. This was a rare moment of intimacy and one of great meaning to Anna. The next day her husband was again irate, but she was much less upset.

I was moved by other ways in which Anna sought to have a meaningful impact, despite the restrictions in her life. One week, for example, she told me she was purchasing a book of elementary Polish so that she could try out a few sentences on a depressed Polish immigrant acquaintance whose mastery of English was poor. "I think hearing me mangle the language will give her a laugh," Anna said. "And she'll know that someone cares."

Anna struggled to reckon with her lack of omnipotence and her illusion of self-sufficiency. Her recognition that she needed household help was a manifestation of this work. She also examined this issue in her relationship with me, exploring her need to control our sessions by taking over, talking, and then telling me when it was my turn. And she developed a sense of humor about her need to control. For example, after a fight with her children about the wording of her own gravestone she was able to say, with a self-deprecating laugh, "I can't believe I've been trying to control what my children will see on my headstone after I'm gone. Maybe it's time for me to let go a bit!"

We have talked about death. Often. As Anna felt the reality of death's approach, she confessed to me her fear of being buried alive. She described in vivid detail what that would be like. I recounted in Chapter 3, the way we came to understand this terror as stemming from the sensory memory of her early months in an incubator and then a hospital. Anna was afraid of the trauma that had already happened – of being isolated and crying fruitlessly with nobody there to hear or comfort. Anna is still afraid of death but no longer preoccupied with fears of being buried alive.

My sessions with Anna exemplify both the pleasure and pain of work with an adult approaching the end of life. As we did the work described earlier, Anna began to feel much better. Despite the hardships in her life – and there were many – she began to enjoy herself. Our sessions were punctuated by laughter. She would tell me about a book she had read, about an old friend who had called, and about finding an item which once belonged to her mother. She consulted me about how to get psychological services for her caregiver's depressed daughter, wanting to help. And one day she told me: "This week I drew the perfect leaf. Truly perfect. It captures the essence of leaf-dom. Now anytime I'm down I can look at it and it gives me joy." Although still suffering, Anna liked herself and was zestfully engaged in life.

This is Chapter 7, "Endings." Earlier in this chapter, I described the various ways the therapies of older adults may conclude and the uncertainty that may attend these conclusions. Sadly, I am living out such an uncertain conclusion with Anna. Recently she contracted Covid-19. She understood that because of her age and medical condition, it was unlikely she would survive. As she was about to leave for the hospital, we talked briefly. Anna said she was frightened. Then, she asked, "Amy, I don't know if you are a person who prays, but if you are, could you please pray for me?" I was moved. At this moment, in Lord's (2019) words, "We are no longer client and psychotherapist. We are two human beings" (p. 137). Although I don't usually pray, I told her I would. (And, yes, I found a way to do that which felt meaningful to me.) We said a hurried goodbye, neither of us knowing if it was for the last time. She was in the hospital and then a rehab facility for weeks. Incredibly, she survived.

Soon after, I call. Her hearing has deteriorated badly and even when wearing hearing aids, she has such difficulty hearing me that after screaming out words repetitively with no success, I resort to spelling them at the top of my lungs. Meanwhile, because my own hearing aids are far from perfect and Anna's voice is uncharacteristically hoarse, I must ask her to repeat herself often. For a minute she is the old Anna, talking with self-deprecating humor about an interaction with a doctor. But she does not hear my response, and soon mental fog drifts in. She is distressed because she does not remember what we are talking about. Continuing in this fashion for more than 10 minutes is exhausting for both of us. Even to discuss whether or how we should/can continue therapy is unworkable. If Covid-19 were not an issue, I would have the option of a home visit. The virus as well as the distance/time involved prevent this. We have agreed to speak next week. Is this an ending? I don't know and I have an ache in my heart.

This work is tough. To work with older adults is to be beset, again and again, with the recognition of human fragility and the brevity of life. It is to face repeated losses of those we grow to love. And it is to recognize that lives (and treatments) end in messy, unpredictable, ways. How do I sustain myself in this work? Partly I do this by the nourishment I find in watching my patients bloom in their later years. But that is not enough.

I am fortunate. I belong to a peer supervision group whose members are a bastion of support, insight, and comfort in dealing with the issues outlined earlier. I also belong to a group of experienced therapists who feel passionate about working with older adults and meet monthly to discuss clinical issues with this age group. In addition, I have several other colleagues with whom I have periodic conversations about the topic. I am not alone. Not every therapist has these resources. Being a therapist to older adults is fulfilling, but it brings pain. As Berzoff (2019) states, "We need to be able to share the suffering with valued colleagues" (p. 126).

I end here with wishes. It is my wish that the community of psychodynamic therapists recognize the value of psychotherapy for older adults and develop its expertise and resources in providing it. It is my wish that as therapists recognize the fulfillment this work offers, many more will undertake it, so that an underserved population receives care. It is my wish that we combat ageism in ourselves, in our patients, and in our society. It is my wish that training programs routinely prepare their candidates to do this work and to recognize the value it offers both patient and therapist. And it is my wish that therapists find creative ways to help each other in this most challenging and rewarding of endeavors.

References

Adelman, A. J. (2013). The hand of fate: On mourning the death of a patient. In A. J. Adelman & K. L. Malawista (Eds.), *The therapist in mourning* (pp. 73–92). Columbia University Press.

Aronson, S. (2009). The (un)designated mourner: When the analyst's patient dies. *Contemporary Psychoanalysis*, *45*(4), 545–560.

Balasubramaniam, M. (2018). Rational suicide in elderly adults: A clinician's perspective. *Journal of the American Geriatrics Society*, *66*(5), 998–1001.

Bergmann, M. S. (2014). Psychoanalysis in old age: The patient and the analyst. In S. Kuchuck (Ed.), *Clinical implications of the psychoanalyst's life experience: When the personal becomes professional* (pp. 237–246). Routledge.

Berzoff, J. (2019). Being still: Sitting with suffering in long-term relational practice. In S. A. Lord (Ed.), *Reflections on long-term relational psychotherapy and psychoanalysis: Relational analysis interminable* (pp. 119–131). Routledge.

Boss, P. (2000). *Ambiguous loss: Learning to live with unresolved grief.* Harvard University Press.

Buechler, S. (2012). *Still practicing: The heartaches and joys of a clinical career.* Routledge.

Buechler, S. (2019). *Psychoanalytic approaches to problems in living: Addressing life's challenges in clinical practice.* Routledge.

Burack-Weiss, A. (2015). *The lioness in winter: Writing an old woman's life.* Columbia University Press.

Daehnert, C. (2008). Crossing over: A story of surrender and transformation. *Contemporary Psychoanalysis*, *44*(2), 199–218.

Freud, S. Letter from Freud to Ludwig Binswanger, April 11, 1929. In *The Sigmund Freud-Ludwig Binswanger correspondence* (1908–1938). Classic Books.

Frommer, M. (2016). Death is nothing at all: On contemplating non-existence. A relational psychoanalytic engagement of the fear of death. *Psychoanalytic Dialogues*, *26*(4), 373–390.

Galatzer-Levy, R. M., & Cohler, B. J. (1990). Chapter 8: The self objects of the second half of life: An introduction. *Progress in Self Psychology*, *6*, 93–109.

Gerson, M-J. (2018). Death of a parent: Openings at an ending. *Psychoanalytic Perspectives*, *15*(3), 340–354.

Hagman, G. (Ed.). (2016). *New models of bereavement theory and treatment: New mourning.* Routledge.

Hoffman, I. Z. (1998). *Ritual and spontaneity in the psychoanalytic process: A dialectical-constructivist view.* Analytic Press.

Horwitz, L. (2005). The capacity of forgive: Intrapsychic and developmental perspectives. *Journal of the American Psychoanalytic Association, 53*(2), 485–511.

Hunter, J. (1999). Panic attacks late in life and change before life ends. *Psychoanalytic Psychotherapy, 13*(3), 233–244.

Lord, S. A. (2019). Till death do us part: Relational work and terminal illness. In S. A. Lord (Ed.), *Reflections on long-term relational psychotherapy and psychoanalysis: Relational analysis Interminable* (pp. 132–140). Routledge.

Marshall, K. (2008). Treating mourning – Knowing loss. *Contemporary Psychoanalysis, 44*(2), 219–233.

Notman, M. T. (2014). Reflections on widowhood and its effects on the self. *Psychodynamic Psychiatry, 42*(1), 65–88.

Peskin, H. (2019). Who has the right to mourn?: Relational deference and the ranking of grief. *Psychoanalytic Dialogues, 29*(4), 477–492.

Quindoz, D. (2010). *Growing old: A journey of self-discovery* (D. Alcorn, Trans.). Routledge (Original work published 2008).

Richards, A. K. (2013). Little boy lost. In A. J. Adelman & K. L. Malawista (Eds.), *The therapist in mourning* (pp. 92–106). Columbia University Press.

Silverman, S. (2010). Will you remember me: Termination and continuity. In J. Salberg (Ed.), *Good enough endings: Breaks, interruptions and terminations from contemporary relational perspectives*. Routledge.

Slochower, J. A. (1993). Mourning and the holding function of shiva. *Contemporary Psychoanalysis, 29*, 352–367.

Tillman, J., & Carter, A. (2014). The trauma of patient suicide. In R. A. Deutsch (Ed.), *Traumatic ruptures: Abandonment and betrayal in the analytic relationship*. Routledge.

Index

For Product Safety Concerns and Information please contact our EU
representative GPSR@taylorandfrancis.com
Taylor & Francis Verlag GmbH, Kaufingerstraße 24, 80331 München, Germany

9 780367 756444